AN ATLAS OF
NORMAL VERTEBRAL
ANGIOGRAMS

AN ATLAS OF NORMAL VERTEBRAL ANGIOGRAMS

PAUL ROSS

M.B., B.S.

Professor and Chairman, Department of Radiology,
Medical University of South Carolina, Charleston, South Carolina, U.S.A.

and

GEORGE H. DU BOULAY

M.B., B.S., F.R.C.P., F.R.C.R.

Professor of Neuroradiology, National Hospital, Queen Square,
London; Radiological Advisor to the Nuffield Institute of
Comparative Medicine, Zoological Society of London.

BUTTERWORTHS

LONDON · BOSTON
Sydney – Wellington – Durban – Toronto

LQM FCH

THE BUTTERWORTH GROUP

ENGLAND

Butterworth & Co (Publishers) Ltd
London: 88 Kingsway, WC2B 6AB

AUSTRALIA

Butterworths Pty Ltd
Sydney: 586 Pacific Highway, NSW 2067
Also at Melbourne, Brisbane, Adelaide
and Perth

SOUTH AFRICA

Butterworth & Co (South Africa) (Pty) Ltd
Durban: 152–154 Gale Street

NEW ZEALAND

Butterworths of New Zealand Ltd
Wellington: 26–28 Waring Taylor Street, 1

CANADA

Butterworth & Co (Canada) Ltd
Toronto: 2265 Midland Avenue,
    Scarborough, Ontario, M1P 4S1

USA

Butterworths (Publishers) Inc
Boston: 161 Ash Street,
    Reading Mass, 01867

First published 1976

ISBN 0 407 00042 9

© Butterworth & Co (Publishers) Ltd 1976

Library of Congress Cataloging in Publication Data

Ross, Paul, 1927–
    An atlas of normal vertebral angiograms.

    Includes bibliographical references.
    1. Cranial fossa, Posterior—Blood vessels—
Atlases. I. du Boulay, G. H., joint author.
II. Title. [DNLM: 1. Cranial fossa, posterior—
Radiography—Atlases. 2. Diencephalon—
Radiography—Atlases. WE17 R825a]
QM455.R67   611'.711   75–34277
ISBN 0 407 00042 9

Printed and bound in Great Britain by
Butler & Tanner Ltd, Frome and London

PREFACE

Vertebral angiography is used increasingly in the diagnosis of lesions involving the posterior cranial fossa and diencephalon, because more accurate interpretation has become possible, based on meticulous studies of the normal anatomy of the posterior fossa arteries and veins and their displacements in disease. The work has been mainly a neuroradiological contribution, many of the vessels not having been described previously by anatomists. Diagnostic difficulties are due not only to the complex arrangement of the vessels in this quite small space, but also to the great number of anatomic variations. This atlas of normal vertebral angiograms is compiled in the hope that illustrating the more common variants will be helpful to neurologists, neurosurgeons and those radiologists who are not expert in the field.

The introductory section assumes only a basic knowledge of the gross anatomy of the relevant parts of the brain. We have not felt it necessary to discuss the anatomy of the vessels in great detail or to compile an extensive bibliography, but references are given to those works which are most helpful in providing the reader with more detailed information. The course of the vessels is described and the segments of each are labelled on the illustrations. Not all the tributaries which have been named by researchers are indicated in the atlas, but we believe that a three dimensional understanding of the course, relationships and variations of those selected is adequate for diagnostic purposes. Finally, it must be emphasized that there are many cases in which some of the opacified vessels, particularly in the venous phase, cannot be confidently identified and a putative set of displacements must make sense anatomically to lead to a tenable diagnosis.

Since making this Atlas, with the assistance of Dr Keller, we have established the mean positions and linear relationships of many of the posterior fossa vascular landmarks, together with their statistical variation. These measurements are given in a paper by Ross, du Boulay and Keller (1975)[47].

PAUL ROSS
GEORGE DU BOULAY

ARTERIES

Vertebral artery

The vertebral artery[7] usually arises from the subclavian artery and is its first branch. After a short upward course it enters the foramen transversarium of C6 and passes vertically through successive foramina transversaria to the level of C2, the foramen transversarium of which is directed laterally as well as upwards. The artery therefore passes laterally and very slightly forward and ascends through the foramen transversarium of C1. Turning sharply medially again and posteriorly, it curves upward and forward, piercing the atlanto-occipital membrane to enter the skull at the lateral margin of the foramen magnum, lying lateral to the medulla. It then passes upward, medially and forward to join the artery of the opposite side, usually near the lower border of the pons, forming the basilar artery. Variations in the course of the vertebral artery are exhaustively reviewed by Krayenbühl[7].

In about three-quarters of cases the left vertebral artery is equal in size to or larger than the right[20]. In the frontal projection the sharp lateral curvature at C2 and medial curvature at C1 are constant features. The intracranial portion of the vertebral artery may appear straight or show marked tortuosity, even in young people. It may pass vertically to the cerebellopontine angle cistern[2] and then turn sharply medially to join its fellow on either side of the midline. At pneumoencephalography it may then produce a density in the cistern which could be mistaken for a tumour. If the two vertebral arteries do not join at the ponto-medullary junction, they more commonly join lower rather than higher[7].

The intracranial portion of the vertebral artery may be narrower than its lower part. The artery may not join the opposite one, but terminate in the posterior inferior cerebellar artery, or its connection to the other vertebral artery may be very narrow.

In the lateral projection one sees the sharp posterior curve of the artery at the level of C1 after it has passed through that transverse foramen and the very acute anterior angulation as it pierces the atlanto-occipital membrane above the posterior arch of the atlas. The intracranial portion may look tortuous, but less so than in the frontal projections, as a rule.

Depending on the length of the extracranial portion of the vertebral artery included on the films, a variable number of *muscular branches* are shown both in frontal and lateral projections. The *anterior meningeal branch*[13] usually arises just below the lateral bend of the vertebral artery at the level of C2, passes medially through the intervertebral foramen and then medially and upwards in the anterior portion of the spinal canal to the level of the foramen magnum where it ends in tiny dural twigs. It can be identified in about half of technically satisfactory vertebral angiograms using the subtraction technique. In the frontal projection, if there is good opacification of both vertebral arteries, the anterior meningeal branches are usually seen to be symmetrical. Except for the most proximal portion, they lie inside the spinal canal, approaching the midline and are slightly tortuous. In the lateral projection a variable portion of the lower two-thirds of the anterior meningeal artery is obscured by the vertebral and the part visualized lies just behind the body of C2 and the odontoid process and in front of the anterior spinal artery. At the C1 level the distal portion is projected in front of the vertebral artery and ends at the anterior margin of the foramen magnum.

The *posterior meningeal branch*[4] arises from the upper margin of the vertebral artery after it has passed over the posterior arch of the atlas and through the atlanto-occipital membrane. It courses upward, backward and medially, entering the dura at the lateral margin of the foramen magnum and, passing to the midline, extends superiorly in the falx cerebelli to the tentorium cerebri. Terminal twigs pass supratentorially into the falx cerebri and adjacent dura. In the frontal projection its proximal portion, which is somewhat tortuous, is seen coursing upward and medially from the superior aspect of the upper horizontal limb of the extracranial vertebral artery, reaching the midline and overlapping the basilar artery. Its distal portion if opacified runs straight upwards near the midline. In the lateral projection it is seen in the space between the sharp anterior loop of the vertebral artery and occipital bone where it may be quite tortuous. It then passes backward and upward following the contour of the occipital bone and lying close to it for a variable distance, usually becoming indiscernible before it has reached the internal occipital protuberance.

The *anterior spinal artery*[5, 35] which lies in the anterior median fissure along the whole length of the spinal cord arises from two branches given off the vertebral arteries 1–3 cm before they join to form the basilar artery. These branches usually unite intracranially but may remain separate, when they are usually connected by anastomoses. Occasionally the origin consists of a single artery. With good technique, the anterior spinal artery can be seen in up to half of normal cases in the lateral projection, lying 1–9 mm behind the posterior margin of the vertebral bodies at the C2 level[5]. It is not tortuous. The subtraction technique is useful for showing it in the frontal projection, where it is visualized less frequently.

The *posterior spinal artery*[6] may be single or paired, lying near the midline on the posterior aspect of the spinal cord. It may arise from the vertebral artery or from the posterior inferior cerebellar artery and also sends a small branch upwards on the posterior aspect of the medulla. The posterior spinal artery has not been identified in normal cases in the frontal projection and can only occasionally be seen in lateral views as a straight vessel near the posterior margin of the spinal canal.

Posterior inferior cerebellar artery[32]

The posterior inferior cerebellar artery (P.I.C.A.) follows a long and tortuous course during which it is related to the medulla, fourth ventricle, cerebellar tonsil, vermis and cerebellar hemisphere so that displacement or distortion of these structures may be deduced from careful study of this artery. Unfortunately, more than any other artery in the posterior fossa, it is subject to many normal variations which may cause diagnostic difficulties. Somewhat different terminology has been employed by various authors[19, 32, 40, 44] and we use that of Huang[37].

In 75–90 per cent of cases the P.I.C.A. originates from the intracranial portion of the vertebral artery, usually 1–2 cm below the basilar artery. It passes downward and laterally along the anterior margin of the medulla but often then loops laterally and upwards before returning to the lateral margin of the medulla. This is the *anterior medullary segment*. The vessel then passes downward around the lateral margin of the medulla forming the anterior and inferior portions of the caudal loop medial to the tonsil, the *lateral medullary segment*. This loop is very variable in its length and occasionally extends below the inferior pole of the tonsil; at other times the lateral medullary segment may pass almost directly backwards. The P.I.C.A. then turns upward and medially to lie behind the posterior surface of the medulla, medial to the tonsil. This is the *posterior medullary segment* and forms the ascending limb of the caudal loop. Continuing upward near the midline, the vessel turns posteriorly near the upper pole of the tonsil where it lies just behind the posterior medullary velum of the fourth ventricle, to become the *supratonsillar segment*. More often than not this segment passes backward medial to the upper pole of the tonsil, but it may course laterally or over the top of it. This segment forms the cranial loop, continuing downward and slightly backward behind the tonsil as the *retrotonsillar segment*, usually several millimetres lateral to the midline, to reach the copula pyramidis which is the ridge connecting the pyramidal lobule of the vermis with the biventral lobule. Here at the copular point the P.I.C.A. turns backward as the *inferior vermian segment* and follows the vermis backward and upward for a variable distance near the midline anastomosing with the terminal branches of the superior vermian artery.

The first and largest branch of the P.I.C.A. is the *tonsillo-hemispheric*, which may be larger than the continuation of the main artery. Hence, some authors describe P.I.C.A. as dividing into a medial and a lateral branch, the medial being the various segments described above and the lateral the tonsillo-hemispheric branch. It arises most commonly from the upper (distal) portion of the posterior medullary segment and runs down again around the tonsil, parallel with and lateral to this segment. However, it continues further downward behind the tonsil and then turns laterally and backward over the cerebellar hemisphere as the *hemispheric branch* which soon divides into two or more smaller branches. As it nears the lower pole of the

2

tonsil the tonsillo-hemispheric branch sends a small tributary forward, the *tonsillar branch*, to supply the lower portion of the tonsil.

One or two very small choroidal branches arise from the anterior half of the supratonsillar segment and run upward and forward to the choroid plexus of the fourth ventricle.

A small artery arises from the vermian segment and runs upward and forward in the fissure behind the pyramidal lobule.

There are innumerable variations in the blood supply of the inferior cerebellum. Sometimes the anterior and posterior inferior cerebellar arteries arise as a common branch from the lower portion of the basilar artery. In such case the P.I.C.A. will often separate as the common stem passes over the anterior surface of the lower part of the pons, the P.I.C.A. then passes downward, medially and backward to reach the posterior margin of the medulla and continue as the posterior medullary segment. Occasionally the lateral medullary segment continues backward either lateral to the tonsil or below it. The tonsillar branch may arise from any portion of the P.I.C.A. proximal to the copula, as a separate artery. Occasionally, the tonsillo-hemispheric branch arises more distally than usual and courses downward and backward over the medial or lateral surface of the tonsil.

In the frontal half-axial projection the anterior medullary segment is usually somewhat tortuous, looping laterally. The lateral medullary segment (the portion which actually relates to the side of the medulla) is short and lies lower than the anterior medullary segment and usually more medial than the most lateral extension of this part of the artery. The posterior medullary segment is long and passes upward. The most medial portion usually lies within 5 mm of the midline and very occasionally a few mm across it. The supratonsillar segment is shorter and usually lies near the midline unless it passes over the lateral surface of the upper pole of the tonsil. The retrotonsillar segment often forms a loop laterally and passes slightly downward and then returns upward and medially to become the inferior vermian segment usually just on its own side of the midline. Occasionally, it passes across so that the inferior vermian segments of both P.I.C.A.s lie just on the same side.

In the straight antero-posterior projection the appearances are similar but the segments of the artery are foreshortened. The lateral medullary segment forms a more distinct downward loop.

In the lateral view the P.I.C.A.s on both sides are demonstrated if reflux down the opposite vertebral artery is achieved. The course of each P.I.C.A. can be followed by examining serial films, since opacification persists longer on the ipsilateral side as a rule. Other distinguishing features are the size, position and branching pattern of each artery, shown on the frontal views. The anterior medullary segment often forms a short

upward loop just behind the vertebral arteries and then passes downward and slightly backward to become the lateral medullary segment which forms the caudal loop. This is very variable in position, but lies above the foramen magnum in 80 per cent of cases. If it is lower, the P.I.C.A. can usually be seen to have a low origin or is very tortuous, and the descending and ascending limbs are close together. These features help to distinguish an anatomical variant from tonsillar herniation. The posterior medullary segment forms the ascending limb of this loop and may pass slightly forward or backward in its upward course. Superiorly it forms the anterior limb of the cranial loop as it curves backward to join the supratonsillar segment This also lies at a variable height[39]. The most antero-superior point of the curve formed by the junction of the posterior medullary and supratonsillar segments has been designated by Huang[37] as the '*choroidal point*'. He measured its position along a line drawn from the anterior margin of the foramen magnum to the torcular. In 50 normal adult angiograms a perpendicular to this line through the choroidal point fell on the average 1 mm behind the junction of the anterior and middle thirds of this line and 90 per cent of the choroidal points were within 2 mm of the average position. It is important to note that in those cases where the course of the artery is anomalous, a choroidal point may not be identifiable in the lateral view, and even if the configuration in this projection is not anomalous, the measurement cannot be relied upon if the junction of the posterior medullary and supratonsillar segments is not near the midline in the frontal view.

The supratonsillar segment curves backward, forming the cranial loop, the descending limb of which, the retrotonsillar segment, passes downward behind the tonsil until it turns sharply backward again around the copula pyramidis where it becomes the inferior vermian segment. The most antero-inferior point on this curve is called the '*copular point*'. Its position along the previously described line has been measured by Huang in a study of the inferior vermian vein which makes the same curve[24], and is described in that section. The inferior vermian artery passes backward and upward, often with gentle undulations about 1 cm from the inner table of the occiput. Occasionally, it can be identified beyond the postero-inferior portion of the vermis where it turns upward and forward, paralleling the straight sinus.

In the lateral view the tonsillo-hemispheric branch may appear to pass downwards next to the posterior medullary segment or it may follow the course of the main artery but passes below the level of the copula pyramidis, in which case it continues as the hemispheric branch near the occipital bone for a variable distance and then sometimes passes upward and backward appearing to cross the inferior vermian artery. A small tonsillar branch may be seen running forward from the inferior retrotonsillar portion of the artery. At other times the tonsillo-hemispheric branch follows an oblique course intermediate between those just described. The choroidal branch is sometimes not visualized, but can often be recognized as a fine tortuous twig passing upward and forward from the anterior part of the supratonsillar segment.

Essence

When the P.I.C.A. is very tortuous or anomalous in position or branching pattern, its distribution can be worked out by remembering that it supplies the vermis by its medial stem which is the main artery for purpose of nomenclature, even though it may be the smaller division. This must pass around the brain stem and terminate near the midline on the inferior vermis, though between these regions the course of the artery is quite variable. The lateral stem, the tonsillo-hemispheric branch supplies the surface of the cerebellar hemisphere and its terminal portion will therefore lie far laterally in the frontal view and close to the occiput preterminally in the lateral view wherever it arises and even if there is more than one such branch. By correlating the position of the various portions of the artery on the frontal and lateral view one can usually determine whether the arrangement is possible anatomically or whether it must be the result of displacement. This is not to say, of course, that every pathological displacement puts the artery into a position which is beyond the limits of anatomic variation.

Basilar artery

The basilar artery is formed by the junction of the two vertebral arteries near the lower margin of the pons. It passes upward on the anterior surface of the pons into the interpeduncular cistern where it bifurcates into its two terminal branches—the posterior cerebral arteries. In the half axial projection the basilar artery is foreshortened; it is better seen in the straight antero-posterior projection. Even in children it is often tortuous and then the proximal or mid-portion is usually further from the midline than the point of terminal bifurcation. Most often the curvature is away from the larger vertebral artery. In the lateral projection the artery tends to curve anteriorly and lies very close to the clivus at the mid-pontine level, but the distance between the anterior margin of the artery and the adjacent clivus is variable. There is even greater variability in this measurement at other points along the course of the artery. The upper portion of the artery often curves posteriorly in the interpeduncular fossa[1]. The termination may be at the level of the upper margin of the dorsum sellae, or above or below this. Rarely it may extend so high as to impinge on the floor of the third ventricle[1]. The upper end of the artery may

be obscured by the proximal posterior cerebral arteries which are seen end-on as they pass laterally. Variations in the course of the basilar artery are extensively reviewed by Krayenbühl[7].

The basilar artery gives rise to the anterior inferior cerebellar arteries, sometimes the internal auditory artery, the pontine arteries, the superior cerebellar arteries and the posterior cerebral arteries.

Anterior inferior cerebellar artery

This usually originates from the lateral side of the lower third of the basilar artery. It passes laterally and slightly downward in the pontine cistern to the 7th and 8th nerves which it accompanies laterally into the cerebello-pontine angle cistern. Typically, the internal auditory artery arises as a small branch just medial to the internal auditory meatus and passes into it with these nerves. Thereafter the anterior inferior cerebellar artery often forms a loop in the cerebello-pontine angle cistern and then divides into two major branches. The *medial branch* travels downward over the biventral lobule of the cerebellum to anastomose with branches of the posterior inferior cerebellar artery. The *lateral branch* loops around the flocculus and then courses laterally near the horizontal fissure of the cerebellum, anastomosing with branches of the superior cerebellar artery over the superior semilunar lobule and with those of the posterior inferior cerebellar artery over the inferior semilunar lobule.

Thirty different types of anomalies of the two anterior inferior cerebellar arteries have been recorded and these are at least as common as the standard arrangement[7]. In 10–25 per cent of patients the posterior inferior cerebellar artery on one side arises from a common trunk with the anterior inferior cerebellar from the proximal portion of the basilar artery.

The following anomalies in the origin of the anterior inferior cerebellar arteries each occur in about 5 per cent of cases. It may make, as just described, a common trunk with the posterior inferior cerebellar artery from the vertebral artery on one side; it may arise together with the posterior inferior cerebellar arteries from the basilar artery on both sides; it may be the terminal branch of a hypoplastic vertebral artery or it may form some combination of the previously described anomalies[8].

As the hemispheric branches of the anterior and posterior inferior cerebellar arteries anastomose freely, there is some variation in the amount of cerebellum supplied by each and the size of the parent arterial trunks tend to be inversely related.

In the frontal view, whether taken in the half-axial or straight antero-posterior projection, the pontine portion of the artery usually shows an inferior convexity. It is often tortuous if the basilar artery curves ipsilaterally. More laterally the artery tends to be tortuous, often looping near the internal auditory meatus. The internal auditory branch is very rarely identifiable. The medial branch, which is usually the smaller, is very foreshortened in the astero-posterior projection but can often be seen passing downward in the half-axial projection. The larger lateral branch can frequently be followed near the upper margin of the petrous temporal bone, its terminal portion passing upward in the half-axial view. Subtraction is needed to visualize it in the straight antero-posterior projection. The inferior loop under the flocculus may be apparent.

In the lateral projection, using the subtraction technique, the main trunk of the artery passes backward and downward continuing as the lateral branch. The medial branch is occasionally seen.

At autopsy the internal auditory artery arose from the basilar artery just above the anterior inferior cerebellar artery in 13–37 per cent[6, 40] of the brains examined, but it is only occasionally demonstrated at angiography usually in the straight antero-posterior projection using subtraction. It passes downward and laterally to the 7th and 8th nerves and accompanies them through the internal auditory meatus. Sometimes it gives off a branch to the lower surface of the cerebellum.

There are 12–20 very small *pontine arteries*[17] arising from the lateral margin of the basilar artery on each side. The medial group, comprising about half, enter the substance of the pons rapidly and are not visualized angiographically. The lateral pontine arteries pass to the lateral margin of the pons before penetrating it and the larger of these are seen as punctate densities projected through the basilar artery in the lateral view. Sometimes the lateral pontine artery near the 5th nerve is larger than the others and it may be projected just in front of the basilar artery. It also sends branches to the nerve and is called the trigeminal artery.

Superior cerebellar artery[9]

The superior cerebellar artery arises from the basilar artery just below its bifurcation and is the most constant of the cerebellar arteries. The main trunk of the artery, which is often duplex[9], is the *circum-mesencephalic portion* and this continues and terminates as the *superior vermian segment*. The named branches are the antero-lateral marginal, hemispheric and precentral cerebellar arteries.

From its origin in the interpeduncular cistern, the artery passes laterally and usually downward over the pons, or it may course through the crural cistern. The emerging 3rd nerve separates the interpeduncular portion from the posterior cerebral artery above. The superior cerebellar artery then turns sharply posteriorly, through the ambient cistern alongside the 4th nerve and also upward to lie adjacent to the midbrain again,

above the brachium conjunctivum and below the free edge of the tentorium. Passing further posteriorly and medially around the midbrain the circum-mesencephalic segment enters the quadrigeminal cistern anteriorly or it may course obliquely over the antero-superior margin of the cerebellum to reach the posterior part of the cistern. It then continues backward over the culmen to become the superior vermian segment, lying near the midline.

At the apex of the cerebellum it turns downward and backward almost at a right-angle and terminates over the declive as fine twigs which anastomose with the distal branches of the inferior vermian segment of the posterior inferior cerebellar artery.

The largest branch is the *antero-lateral marginal artery* which usually arises from the ambient portion of the circum-mesencephalic segment. It passes forward and laterally toward the anterior angle of the cerebellum and the horizontal fissure along which it continues posteriorly to anastomose with hemispheric branches of the inferior cerebellar arteries.

Two or three *hemispheric branches* arise from the posterior portion of the circum-mesencephalic segment and pass upward over the antero-superior margin of the cerebellum on to its superior surface and then downward, laterally and posteriorly towards the horizontal fissure.

The *precentral cerebellar arteries* are small branches arising from the anterior culminate portion of the superior vermian artery. They pass forward and downward into the precentral cerebellar fissure. At the level of the inferior colliculi they turn backward to run just behind and parallel to the roof of the upper part of the 4th ventricle and enter the cerebellum at the lower end of the precentral cerebellar fissure.

In the frontal half-axial projection the proximal superior cerebellar arteries are projected below the posterior cerebral arteries, often lower on one side than the other. They turn sharply posteriorly and medially, crossing the image of the posterior cerebral arteries at or just behind the point where these turn backwards. They then run parallel to or diverge medially from them. Tortuous proximally, the superior vermian segments pass upward and slightly medially and at the apex of the cerebellum curve abruptly downward as thin straight vessels to fade out, or sometimes join the inferior vermian segments of the posterior inferior cerebellar artery. The arteries are considerably foreshortened in the straight antero-posterior view.

The antero-lateral marginal branch passes laterally, usually with a downward convexity and only mild tortuosity, often partly overlapped by middle and anterior temporal branches of the posterior cerebral artery in the half-axial projection. It then turns quite sharply upwards as it reaches the lateral angle of the cerebellum. In the straight antero-posterior view it is foreshortened but can be identified on subtraction films, coursing below the temporal branches of the posterior cerebral artery, often symmetrically on each side.

The hemispheric branches are often difficult to see in the half-axial projection as they pass laterally and posteriorly in the same direction as the larger temporal branches of the posterior cerebral artery and this difficulty is compounded in the antero-posterior view.

The precentral cerebellar arteries are not seen in frontal projections.

Unless the basilar artery terminates unusually low, the lateral mesencephalic portion of the superior cerebellar artery curves downward in the lateral view. As it passes posteriorly it is overlapped by the posterior temporal branches of the posterior cerebral arteries. Their internal occipital segments overlap the anterior culminate portions of the superior vermian arteries but these can be identified around the cerebellar apex at or just above the level of the posterior cerebral arteries by their characteristic right-angle turn and then followed downward and backward for a variable distance. The hemispheric branches are usually recognizable lying almost parallel to the terminal superior vermian artery and in front of it. In subtraction views the antero-lateral marginal branch can be seen curving downward, forward in its proximal portion and then backward, sometimes down to the horizontal fissure. The precentral cerebellar arteries, or the largest branch, can sometimes be identified by the almost vertically downward course with a slight anterior convexity to the level of the inferior colliculi, but rarely much further.

Posterior cerebral artery

The posterior cerebral artery[44] originates from the terminal bifurcation of the basilar artery. Its circummesencephalic portion passes around the midbrain in the interpeduncular, crural, ambient and quadrigeminal cisterns near the tentorium and becomes the internal occipital segment as it crosses the free edge of the tentorial notch to lie on the medial aspect of the occipital lobe. It divides into its terminal parietooccipital and calcarine branches at a variable point along its course. The named branches are the thalamoperforate, medial and lateral posterior choroidal splenial and anterior, middle and posterior temporal arteries.

Passing from its origin in the interpeduncular cistern around the cerebral peduncle above the 3rd nerve through the crural cistern, the *circum-mesencephalic segment* curves backward with a downward convexity around the midbrain. In the ambient cistern it lies medial to the hippocampal gyrus, above and slightly lateral to the superior cerebellar artery. As it reaches the quadrigeminal cistern it courses medially and upward towards the calcarine fissure below the splenium of the corpus callosum medial to the antero-superior portion of the lingual gyrus. It may bifurcate into its terminal branches at any point beyond the crural cistern.

Six to twelve *thalamoperforate arteries*[10, 22] arise from the upper end of the basilar artery and the adjacent portions of the posterior cerebral arteries. They pass upward and backward through the interpeduncular cistern to enter the posterior perforated substance and then upward and slightly laterally into the diencephalon. About 1 cm from its origin, the posterior cerebral artery is connected to the supraclinoid portion of the internal carotid artery by the *posterior communicating artery* which passes forward and slightly laterally with a mild downward convexity from the interpeduncular through the chiasmatic cistern. It gives rise to a few *anterior thalamoperforate arteries* which pass upward and posteriorly into the base of the brain lateral to the mamillary body, branching to supply the anterior thalamic region.

The *medial posterior choroid artery*[11] arises from the proximal posterior cerebral artery in the interpeduncular or crural cistern. It runs around the brain stem in the ambient cistern, just medial to the posterior cerebral artery and then into the quadrigeminal cistern where it turns sharply forward to pass upward and medially, lying just lateral to the pineal body. As it reaches the level of the anterior margin of the pineal it curves backward again and courses upward to reach the roof of the 3rd ventricle near the midline which it follows forward, supplying the choroid plexus.

There are usually two lateral *posterior choroid arteries*[11], both arising from the ambient portion of the posterior cerebral artery. The more anterior one, which is usually small, curves antero-laterally in the choroid fissure to supply the choroid plexus in the anterior part of the temporal horn, anastomosing with the anterior choroid artery. The larger posterior branch passes backward and laterally in the choroid fissure below the thalamus and usually divides into two branches. The small medial one runs up behind the thalamus to end in the tela choroidea. The larger lateral branch curves forward and laterally around the pulvinar of the thalamus following the choroid plexus of the posterior part of the temporal horn through the trigone into the posterior portion of the body of the lateral ventricle.

The *splenial artery*[44] (posterior pericallosal artery, dorsal callosal artery) arises from the ambient portion of the posterior cerebral artery just behind the lateral posterior choroid arteries. Following the posterior cerebral artery backward it diverges from it in the quadrigeminal cistern and curls around the splenium of the corpus callosum to anastomose with terminal twigs of the pericallosal branch of the anterior cerebral artery.

The *anterior temporal artery* arises as one or more

branches at or just behind the crural segment of the posterior cerebral artery. It courses downward, forward and laterally, anastomosing with anterior temporal branches of the middle cerebral artery on the inferior surface of the anterior portion of the temporal lobe.

A few *middle temporal arteries* originate from the ambient portion of the posterior cerebral artery and pass laterally and downward to the undersurface of the mid-portion of the temporal lobe where they anastomose with corresponding branches of the middle cerebral artery.

In 80 per cent of the cases the *posterior temporal artery* arises as a single trunk usually from the ambient segment of the posterior cerebral artery, occasionally from the quadrigeminal segment. There are two or more trunks of origin in 20 per cent[13]. It courses posteriorly, laterally and slightly downward along the parahippocampal gyrus to the lingual gyrus anastomosing with posterior temporal branches of the middle cerebral artery laterally and inferior branches of the calcarine artery posteriorly.

The *parieto-occipital artery*, the larger of the two terminal branches of the posterior cerebral artery, arises from its internal occipital segment in 40 per cent of cases[13]—in the remainder the bifurcation occurs more proximally and there is then no internal occipital segment. It passes posteriorly and upward over the cingulate gyrus terminating in branches to the precuneus, parieto-occipital fissure and cuneus. It anastomoses with the pericallosal branch of the anterior cerebral artery and with the calcarine artery.

The *calcarine artery* arises as one or two trunks lateral to the parieto-occipital artery. Crossing it on a postero-medial course, it enters the calcarine fissure and is the principal, though often not the only source of blood supply to the visual cortex[14].

In the frontal half-axial projection the proximal parts of the posterior cerebral arteries pass laterally (and downward unless the basilar artery is short), to cross the superior cerebellar arteries and then curve upward lateral to them. Often one artery courses further laterally in the ambient cistern than the other and this asymmetry may be seen in the further course and branching pattern. The arteries approach each other in the quadrigeminal cistern, wander upward for a short distance, about 2 cm apart, and terminate in the larger parieto-occipital artery medially and the calcarine artery laterally. The parieto-occipital artery breaks up into a number of moderately tortuous branches which pass upward more or less vertically whereas the calcarine artery shows fewer branches and crosses the former with a medial and upward inclination. Usually a distinct calcarine branch reaches the midline and passes straight upward. Other branches are superimposed upon those of the parieto-occipital artery.

Sometimes the posterior cerebral artery receives most of its blood from the internal carotid through a large posterior communicating artery, or all if the posterior cerebral artery originates exclusively from the internal carotid artery. On vertebral angiography there is then only momentary opacification of that posterior cerebral artery or it is not visualized at all. Usually some contrast medium enters one or both posterior communicating arteries, which opacify on one or two films at rapid serial angiography, passing downward and laterally 1 cm from the origin of the posterior cerebral artery. Sometimes there is flash filling of the internal carotid artery and its terminal branches.

Thalamo-perforate branches are often seen as very thin tortuous twigs passing upward for a short distance above the origin of the posterior cerebral arteries near the midline. Sometimes the medial choroid artery is visualized as a fine vessel coursing just inside the loop formed by the posterior cerebral artery, but its distal portion which passes to the midline and then straight downward can only rarely be seen. The lateral posterior choroidal artery is usually obscured by the temporal branches of the posterior cerebral artery and hemispheric branches of the superior cerebellar artery, but occasionally the more posterior of the two branches is discernable as a fine twig, passing upward from the ambient portion of the posterior cerebral artery. The anterior temporal branches follow a mildly tortuous course laterally and downward overlapping the antero-lateral marginal branch of the superior cerebellar artery and then the hemispheric branches of the inferior cerebellar arteries. The middle temporal branches, also mildly tortuous, pass laterally and overlap the hemispheric branches of the superior cerebellar artery. The posterior temporal artery usually follows a more tortuous course upward and laterally supplying branches to this portion of the temporal lobe and often middle and even anterior temporal branches. The splenial artery cannot be identified in this projection.

The posterior cerebral artery and its branches are foreshortened in the antero-posterior projection and the smaller ones are not discernible. However, the infratentorial cerebellar branches are projected below the supratentorial temporal branches. The calcarine branches are projected below those of the parieto-occipital artery.

In the lateral view the most proximal portions of the posterior cerebral arteries are usually seen on end as dense shadows but sometimes they swing forward in front of the basilar artery. The ambient portions of the posterior cerebral arteries pass backward with a mild inferior convexity, not as marked as the curvature of the corresponding segments of the superior cerebellar arteries, unless the basilar artery is unusually short when these segments are straight.

The quadrigeminal and internal occipital portions of the posterior cerebral arteries overlap the superior cerebellar arteries as they pass backward and slightly upward, the internal occipital segments usually showing a mild upward convexity. The calcarine branches follow the direction of the main trunks posteriorly while the parieto-occipital branches course above them upward and posteriorly.

The posterior communicating arteries pass forward usually with a downward convexity. The thalamo-perforate arteries in their upward course frequently run first posteriorly with a gentle tortuosity proximally and then a straighter vertical termination. The most proximal horizontal portions of the posterior choroid arteries are obscured by the posterior cerebral arteries. The medial posterior choroid artery then shows a characteristic figure-3 shape as it curves upward and then around the level of the front of the pineal ending, after a second posterior convexity superiorly, in the choroid plexus of the roof of the 3rd ventricle. The lateral posterior choroid arteries lie just behind the medial ones and form a smooth arc ending in the blush of the choroid plexus of the lateral ventricle, which obscures their distal portions. The splenial artery, which lies behind the posterior choroid arteries, is also obscured proximally by the posterior cerebral arteries. It then curves smoothly round the splenium of the corpus callosum diverging from the posterior choroid arteries inferiorly and paralleling them posteriorly and superiorly.

The anterior temporal branches follow a tortuous course downward and forward for a variable distance in front of the basilar artery. The middle temporal branches wind predominantly downward over the superior cerebellar arteries and their more anterior branches. The larger posterior temporal arteries pass obliquely downward and backward over the distal portions of the superior vermian arteries, often obscuring the more posterior hemispheric branches of the superior cerebellar artery.

VEINS

The veins of the posterior fossa and their many variations have been studied in Byzantine detail over the last ten years and only a simplified account is given here, together with references to the more important original papers. The embryology has been carefully studied by Padget[36] and summarized by Krayenbühl[7].

The veins which may be demonstrated on vertebral angiography are situated in the supratentorial as well as the infratentorial region. They are classified on the basis of their drainage into three groups. The anterior group drains into the superior or inferior petrosal sinus, the posterior group drains into the lateral sinus or lower part of the straight sinus and the superior group drains into the great vein of Galen or the upper part of the straight sinus.

The anterior group of veins[15] comprises those related to the front of the brain stem, namely, the anterior ponto-mesencephalic veins, the anterior medullary veins and the transverse pontine veins; those passing forward over the upper and lower surface of the cerebellar hemispheres, namely, some of the superior hemispheric and inferior hemispheric veins, and the vein of the great horizontal fissure, as well as the posterior spinal vein and the retro-olivary vein, the vein of the lateral recess of the 4th ventricle and those brachial veins which run forward to join the petrosal vein.

The posterior group comprises the inferior vermian vein and its retrotonsillar tributaries and many of the superior and inferior hemispheric veins.

The supratentorial veins of the superior group include the superior thalamic vein, the superior choroid vein, the splenial (posterior pericallosal) vein, the basal vein of Rosenthal and inferior occipital veins. The infratentorial veins are the lateral mesencephalic vein, the precentral cerebellar vein and those brachial veins draining into it, the superior vermian vein and the posterior mesencephalic vein and its peduncular tributary.

The *anterior ponto-mesencephalic vein*[16, 23] outlines the interpeduncular fossa and anterior margin of the pons. It usually originates in the region of the anterior perforated substance and passes postero-medially into the depth of the interpeduncular cistern to reach the midline. It then angles sharply forward and passes out of the cistern to run downward on the anterior surface of the pons near the midline. Sometimes it communicates inferiorly with the *anterior medullary vein* which is usually the upward continuation of one or more small veins passing vertically along the anterior surface of the spinal cord. Most often the anterior ponto-mesencephalic vein drains into *transverse pontine veins* which run laterally, more or less horizontally near the midportion of the pons, directly into the petrosal vein or less often into the superior or inferior petrosal sinus or lateral mesencephalic vein. Occasionally, the anterior ponto-mesencephalic vein does not reach the midline but passes downward on one or other cerebral peduncle without entering the interpeduncular cistern and then courses down the antero-lateral margin of the pons. Two or more laterally positioned veins may replace the midline vein.

9

In the frontal half-axial projection the most proximal portions of the vein may be faintly seen forming an inferiorly convex curve as they pass over the cerebral peduncles on each side. The interpeduncular segment passes straight down near the midline to become the pontine segment and then curves to one or other side as it enters a transverse pontine vein. This often shows a curve with an inferior convexity as it passes laterally to the petrosal vein. The anterior medullary vein may be seen as a faint vertical density below this level.

In the lateral view the characteristic sharp turn as the anterior ponto-mesencephalic vein reverses direction in the floor of the interpeduncular cistern is usually evident. The anteriorly convex pontine segment can be followed down behind the clivus for a variable distance and in subtraction films the anterior medullary vein is occasionally seen continuous with it. The transverse pontine vein is foreshortened, but may be seen passing backward, often mildly tortuous.

Some of the *superior* and *inferior hemispheric veins* drain anteriorly, passing along the named cerebellar fissures or across the lobules of the cerebellum. They may empty directly into the petrosal sinuses or the petrosal vein. Sometimes the superior hemispheric veins join a transverse channel, the antero-lateral marginal vein, which passes medially along that border of the cerebellum into the petrosal vein. Not infrequently there is an identifiable *vein of the great horizontal fissure* which runs anteriorly, at first slightly laterally from the depth of the fissure and then turns medially on to the anterior surface of the lower portion of the cerebellar hemisphere and upward to join the petrosal vein. It usually receives some of the inferior hemispheric veins.

In the frontal half-axial projection the superior hemispheric veins run downward with a mild lateral convexity toward the petrous temporal bone, the inferior hemispheric veins run upward toward it. The vein of the great horizontal fissure passes downward and laterally and curves abruptly medially forming an acute angle to pass more or less horizontally to the petrosal vein.

In the lateral view the superior hemispheric veins course obliquely downward and forward, the inferior hemispheric veins upward and forward. The vein of the great horizontal fissure passes forward with a gentle downward convexity, turning upward near its termination.

One or more vertical venous channels lie behind the cervical spinal cord. These are the *posterior spinal veins* which drain upward into the veins on the posterior and lateral aspect of the medulla. The more medial of the retromedullary veins is the vein of the restiform body which follows this structure upward and laterally. Running upward and along the lateral margin of the medulla is the *retro-olivary vein* which turns abruptly laterally near the ponto-medullary junction to join either the lateral pontine vein or the vein of the lateral recess of the 4th ventricle.

In the frontal half-axial projection the retro-olivary vein may be seen passing upward from the region of the anterior margin of the foramen magnum and slightly laterally almost up to the level of the petrosal vein where it curls sharply laterally toward it.

In the lateral view the posterior spinal vein may occasionally be seen in the upper cervical region but the retro-olivary vein can rarely be identified.

Huang[47] discovered a paired vein draining anteriorly which bears a constant relationship to the 4th ventricle and named it the *vein of the lateral recess of the 4th ventricle*, abbreviated V.L.R. It arises from veins draining the upper pole of the tonsil and passes forward, laterally and downward just below the lateral recess of the 4th ventricle to the cerebello-ponto-medullary angle. Here it turns laterally below the flocculus and then upward, forward and medially usually between the brachium pontis and the cerebellar hemisphere to reach the anterior angle of the hemisphere, that is, the junction of the antero-superior and antero-lateral margins, where it is joined by the other veins which drain into the petrosal vein. Often the V.L.R. drains directly into the inferior or superior petrosal sinus so that the distal portion is absent.

In the frontal half-axial view the proximal, medial portion of the V.L.R. starts about 12 mm from the midline and passes downward and laterally, often with a slight lateral convexity to a point just medial to the internal auditory meatus. Characteristically it then curves back upward and medially, paralleling its proximal portion and enters the petrosal vein which may be superimposed on it.

In the lateral view the proximal part of the V.L.R. passes forward and slightly downward, overlapped by the posterior mastoid air cells, at a level just below the external auditory meatus. Using subtraction the portion of the vein passing under the flocculus may be seen angling sharply upward and then also forward.

A number of paired veins pass along the upper surface of the brachium conjunctivum and brachium pontis, some draining upward and posteriorly, others downward and anteriorly. These are called *brachial veins*. Those draining anteriorly may lie deep, or superficially near the antero-superior margin of the cerebellum and they pass laterally and slightly downward to join the anteriorly draining veins of the superior and inferior surface of the cerebellar hemisphere, the vein of the horizontal fissure, the antero-lateral marginal vein, the transverse pontine vein and the V.L.R. to form the *petrosal vein* near the anterior angle of the cerebellum. This is a short stem which runs antero-laterally to join the superior petrosal sinus, often just lateral to the internal auditory meatus. Sometimes two or more veins drain into the superior petrosal sinus at different points.

In the frontal half-axial view the brachial vein

passes downward and laterally, sometimes joining the lateral mesencephalic vein superiorly with the petrosal vein inferiorly. The petrosal vein often continues in a direct line with the brachial vein but appears denser and wider because it is more foreshortened and receives contrast medium from the other veins draining into it. If the posterior inferior cerebellar artery on one side is not opacified the petrosal vein usually appears faint or may not be visible, since that artery supplies much of the territory drained by the petrosal vein[45].

In the lateral projection the brachial vein, if visualized, passes forward and slightly downward and the petrosal vein passes forward near the dense shadow of the petrous temporal bones.

The *superior petrosal sinus* passes from the cavernous sinus laterally and posteriorly along the upper margin of the petrous ridge to join the sigmoid sinus. The *inferior petrosal sinus* lies more medially at the postero-inferior margin of the petrous temporal bone and passes posteriorly to join the sigmoid sinus near the jugular foramen.

In the frontal half-axial view the superior petrosal sinus passes laterally and slightly upward, following the upper margin of the petrous temporal bone. Depending upon the precise projection the superior sinus may appear to overlap or ride above the bony margin. The inferior petrosal sinus is not usually seen. In the lateral projection the superior petrosal sinus is foreshortened but a variable portion may be visualized coursing from the upper clivus downward and backward. The inferior petrosal sinus is occasionally shown on subtraction views passing more or less horizontally posteriorly at a lower level.

The most important of the posterior group of veins is the paired *inferior vermian vein*[24]. This originates behind the tonsil at about its midlevel by the junction of the superior and inferior retrotonsillar tributaries. The *superior retrotonsillar tributary* arises from small veins draining the upper pole of the tonsil and runs downward and slightly backward behind the upper half of the tonsil to the copula pyramidis, the ridge connecting the pyramidal lobule of the vermis with the cerebellar hemisphere. There it curls backward and medially to join the inferior vermian vein. The *inferior retrotonsillar tributary* arises a little more laterally from small veins on the undersurface of the cerebellar hemisphere and passes postero-medially to reach the posterior border of the lower portion of the tonsil where it runs upward and slightly backward to join the superior retrotonsillar tributary near the copula pyramidis.

The inferior vermian vein passes from the copula pyramidis backward and upward near the midline along the inferior vermis, demarcating the anterior margin of the cisterna magna and drains into the lower end of the straight sinus. Occasionally it lies more laterally on the medial border of the cerebellar hemisphere and is then lower in position. Sometimes it turns laterally at its distal end and enters the lateral sinus near the torcular. Along its course it is joined by small veins from the inferior surface of the cerebellum.

In the frontal half-axial projection the superior retrotonsillar tributary, which is foreshortened, passes vertically downward a few millimetres from the midline and characteristically hooks abruptly medially to join the inferior vermian vein. The more prominent inferior retrotonsillar tributary passes upward and medially to continue into the inferior vermian vein which courses upward often with a gentle medial convexity near the midline to the region of the torcular.

In the lateral view the superior retrotonsillar tributary passes downward and slightly backward in a straight line to the copula pyramidis where it turns sharply backward and upward. The inferior retrotonsillar tributary runs backward and upward with a gentle posterior convexity to join the inferior vermian vein which courses backward and upward, gradually diverging further from the occipital bone, unless it lies unusually far laterally on the medial portion of the cerebellar hemisphere when it is more inferior in position. Either of the retrotonsillar tributaries may be small or absent. The inferior vermian vein should not be confused with the *occipital sinus* which lies in the midline on the occipital bone and is occasionally visualized, or with inferior hemispheric veins which lie closer to the occipital bone than the inferior vermian vein and more laterally.

Huang and others[24] have defined the 'copular point' for measurement purposes, as the most antero-inferior point of the curve formed by the junction of the superior retrotonsillar tributary and the inferior vermian vein in the lateral view. A line was drawn from the torcular to the anterior margin of the foramen magnum and bisected. The mean position of the copular point was 4 mm behind and 4 mm below the midpoint of the line and in 98 per cent of the 50 normal cases measured, the copular point was within a circle of 6 mm radius from the mean position.

There are *superior* and *inferior hemispheric veins* draining posteriorly, mainly into the transverse sinus and also into the straight sinus. The larger ones tend to run in the cerebellar fissures, and the inferior hemispheric veins are often larger than the superior ones. Sometimes a few hemispheric veins join posteriorly to form a common trunk before joining the sinus and this has been called the posterior cerebellar vein. The hemispheric veins often appear mildly tortuous in the frontal view and tend to have a slight curvature convex laterally. In the lateral view they frequently show up prominently below the inferior vermian veins and may cross them.

Of the supratentorial superior draining group of veins, the *basal vein of Rosenthal*, which is usually, but not always, entirely supratentorial in location[25], is too well known to merit description here. The paired *superior thalamic vein* (postero-medial thalamic vein) is the largest of the veins draining the thalamus, which receives most of its blood supply by the vertebro-basilar system[27]. Occasionally the other much smaller draining tributaries, the inferior and posterior thalamic veins, can be identified but they are unimportant and will not be described.

The superior thalamic vein drains mainly the upper and medial portion of the thalamus. It arises from the union of many small veins coming out on to the medial surface of the thalamus about its midportion. Passing under the fornix downward and backward on the thalamus in the lateral wall of the 3rd ventricle it empties into the posterior end of the internal cerebral vein or into the great vein of Galen.

The paired *superior choroid vein*, which drains the choroid plexus of the trigone and body of the lateral ventricle is the only choroid vein normally visible radiographically in the adult[27]. The inferior choroid vein which drains the temporal horn choroid plexus may be seen in children. Many small veins unite in the region of the trigone to form the superior choroid vein which runs forward, in the lateral wall of the body of the lateral ventricle often at about its midlevel and following the antero-posterior curve of the lateral ventricle empties into the thalamo-striate vein or the anterior end of the internal cerebral vein.

The paired *splenial vein*[43] arises from small twigs passing out of the corpus callosum near its midportion and follows it back close to the midline to enter the posterior end of the great vein of Galen.

The *internal occipital veins* drain the medial and inferior surface of the occipital lobe. They have been named individually according to the gyrus which each drains[28], but this seems unnecessarily complex. Usually two or three venous channels are apparent passing forward more or less horizontally to join the great vein of Galen or the posterior ends of one of the other veins draining into it.

In the frontal view the superior thalamic, superior choroid and splenial veins are foreshortened and over-lapped by larger veins lying near the midline so that they cannot be identified. The internal occipital veins pass downward and slightly medially from above the torcular to the great vein of Galen.

In the lateral projection, the superior thalamic vein is the lowest of the three curved supratentorial veins seen at vertebral angiography. As the arterio-venous circuit in the thalamus is rapid, it appears early in the venous phase and fades before the other veins. It shows the least amount of curvature, convex postero-superiorly and is usually almost straight, 2–3 cm in length and lies just below the internal cerebral vein which is sometimes seen on vertebral angiography. The superior thalamic vein is the most constantly visualized of the three veins, and often the veins on each side can be seen where they do not quite overlap.

The superior choroid vein is seen less often as it is frequently obscured by the blush of the choroid plexus. It lies above the level of the internal cerebral vein, shows a marked curve convex postero-superiorly and runs a longer course. It is typically tortuous from the region of the trigone to the junction of the thalamo-striate and internal cerebral veins, though it may not be visible throughout its entire length.

The splenial vein is sometimes opacified and follows about the same curvature, higher and further posterior-ly, just below the level of the inferior sagittal sinus, which is not shown on vertebral angiography. It is usually 2–3 cm in length.

The internal occipital veins are always shown when the posterior cerebral artery is opacified. They cross the straight sinus, superior vermian and sometimes superior hemispheric veins as they pass more or less horizontally to the region of the great vein of Galen. Their origin behind the straight sinus identifies them as supratentorial veins.

Of the infratentorial superior draining group of veins the most important is the unpaired *precentral cerebellar vein*[30]. It is formed by the junction of two *brachial tributaries*, each originating from small veins on the upper surface of the brachium pontis laterally. Passing backward and medially over it and the brach-ium conjunctivium, the brachial tributary joins its fellow near the midline. At its origin the precentral cerebellar vein therefore lies deep in the precentral fissure on the precentral lobule of the vermis and just behind the lingula and anterior medullary velum which form the roof of the upper part of the 4th ven-tricle. It runs upward and forward on the central lobule near the midline, parallel to the roof of the 4th ven-tricle to the level of the lower margin of the inferior colliculi. Here the vein makes a distinct turn backward as it passes through the upper end of the precentral fissure behind the inferior colliculi to course upward and backward in front of the culmen of the vermis. It continues in this direction through the quadrigeminal cistern to join the posterior part of the great vein of Galen. Variations of the precentral cerebellar vein are not rare. The brachial tributaries may run upward for a variable distance before joining or rarely con-tinue independently to join the posterior ends of the internal cerebral veins. Sometimes the precentral cerebellar vein lies more laterally in the precentral cerebellar fissure and then this portion also lies more anteriorly and continues directly upward and back-ward without the characteristic anteriorly convex bend. Occasionally the precentral cerebellar vein is poorly developed, the brachial veins draining forward and laterally into the petrosal vein. Variations in the distal, upper portion of the precentral cerebellar vein, which may join the superior vermian, internal cerebral or posterior mesencephalic veins near the great vein of Galen are common but unimportant.

In the frontal half-axial projection the precentral cerebellar vein may be obscured by the inferior vermian veins. Usually it passes straight upward in the midline to the great vein of Galen. If it lies paracentrally it may show a gentle curvature convex medially. The brachial veins may be somewhat asymmetrical and pass medially and upward, usually with a mild inferior convexity.

In the lateral view the direction of the lower portion of the precentral cerebellar vein, if it lies in the midline, indicates the slope of the roof of the upper part of the 4th ventricle. The most anterior point of the characteristic knee convex anteriorly, where the vein lies between the inferior colliculi and the precentral lobule, has been designated by Huang and Wolf[30] as the 'colliculo-central point'. In forty presumably normal adult angiograms they found that a line drawn through this point perpendicular to Twining's line was within 5 per cent of the midpoint of that line. Above this region the precentral cerebellar vein courses more or less straight upward and backward. Confusion may arise when there is a superior hemispheric vein with a similar shape. This lies further posteriorly. If the anterior tributary of the superior vermian vein is prominent it may simulate the precentral cerebellar vein, but the former often shows a little scalloping as it passes over the folia of the vermis. In doubtful cases tomography is useful to identify the precentral cerebellar vein.

The paired *lateral mesencephalic vein*[35], shows much variation in its drainage and can therefore be classified as an anterior or a superior draining vein. Wackenheim[34] describes six such variations. Classically, the laterally mesencephalic vein is joined at its lower end by the brachial tributary of the petrosal vein on the brachium pontis. It then passes upward in the lateral mesencephalic sulcus, which is a vertical groove on the lateral aspect of the midbrain between the cerebral peduncle antero-laterally and the tegmentum postero-medially, to drain into the posterior mesencephalic vein or slightly higher into the basal vein of Rosenthal. Occasionally, it drains superiorly into the precentral cerebellar vein. The French workers[34] include the anteriorly draining tributary of the petrosal vein as the inferior portion of the lateral mesencephalic vein, and since this brachial vein may enter the petrosal system by any of the veins which characteristically empty into the petrosal vein many combinations of anterior and superior connections of the lateral mesencephalic vein are obtained. Sometimes the lateral mesencephalic and brachial veins are large, forming a prominent anastomosis between the posterior mesencephalic and petrosal veins and this complex has been called the lateral anastomotic mesencephalic vein.

The paired *posterior mesencephalic vein*[29], which may consist of more than one channel, arises from its *peduncular tributary*[29]. This originates near the midline in the interpeduncular fossa and encircles the cerebral peduncle, thus delineating its contour. The posterior mesencephalic vein may also receive superior tributaries from the adjacent portion of the temporal lobe. Occasionally, it arises from veins passing along the pons or from the lateral mesencephalic vein. It

passes backward and slightly upward around the midbrain and through the quadrigeminal cistern to join the lower part of the vein of Galen or one of its main tributaries. Sometimes it replaces the basal vein, and then it is large[29].

The paired *superior vermian vein*[29] arises from small superior hemispheric tributaries near the junction of the declive and culmen of the vermis. It passes upward and forward over the apex of the cerebellum and then continues forward on the culmen for a short distance, finally curving abruptly upward to enter the lower portion of the vein of Galen. Often it is joined by a smaller anterior superior vermian vein which arises in the fissure between the culmen and the central lobule and follows the border of the culmen upward and backward. Occasionally, the superior vermian and precentral cerebellar veins unite before their termination. If there is only a single midline superior vermian vein, it can be recognized by its larger size.

In the frontal half-axial projection the superior vermian vein is foreshortened and obscured by the straight sinus. The peduncular veins, when visualized, curve laterally with a gentle downward convexity symmetrically from the midline, outlining the cerebral peduncles and join the antero-lateral ends of the posterior mesencephalic veins. The peduncular vein may be confused with a well-developed brachial tributary of the precentral cerebellar vein, connecting it to the lateral mesencephalic vein. This, in the frontal half-axial view, lies at a higher level and its connection to the precentral vein is apparent medially whereas the peduncular vein fades to the limit of visibility here. Bilateral anastomoses between the precentral vein and the lateral mesencephalic veins are very rare. The posterior mesencephalic veins are usually quite wide but not densely opacified. They pass straight upward and medially symmetrically, forming an inverted V, to the vein of Galen. The lateral mesencephalic veins are projected above the peduncular veins, the main trunk running vertically about 15 mm from the midline and its upper portion which is often faint, curving laterally to the posterior mesencephalic vein. Inferiorly it is continuous with the brachial vein which drains into the petrosal vein.

In the lateral view the lateral mesencephalic vein runs vertically in front of the precentral cerebellar vein and enters the posterior mesencephalic vein. The latter are often seen separately one just above the other, following the tentorial notch backward and upward to the vein of Galen in the same direction as the basal vein of Rosenthal which occasionally replaces one of them. The superior vermian vein passes upward and forward diverging from the straight sinus as it approaches the cerebellar apex and terminating in the vein of Galen by coursing forward for about 1 cm and then upward. It may be joined by a small tributary running backward and upward behind the precentral cerebellar vein over the anterior surface of the culmen.

SUMMARY AND REVIEW

It is useful to review the arteries and veins seen on vertebral angiography in terms of the portions of the brain which they demarcate. The *anterior surface of the brain stem* is delineated from below upward by the anterior spinal artery and vein, the distal vertebral artery and the anterior medullary vein, the pontine segment of the anterior inferior cerebellar artery, the basilar and pontine arteries and the pontine segment of the anterior ponto-mesencephalic vein, the proximal portions of the superior cerebellar and posterior cerebral arteries and the thalamo-perforate and proximal medial posterior choroidal arteries, the peduncular portion of the anterior ponto-mesencephalic vein and the peduncular tributary of the posterior mesencephalic vein. The *lateral surface of the brain stem* is not accurately demarcated inferiorly where the related vessels are the vertebral artery after it passes intracranially, the lateral medullary segment of the posterior inferior cerebellar artery, the retro-olivary vein and the proximal portion of the vein of the lateral recess of the 4th ventricle. In the ponto-mesencephalic region the anterior end of the posterior mesencephalic vein, the lateral mesencephalic vein and, less constantly, the ambient portion of the superior cerebellar artery are closely applied to the brain stem. The *posterior surface of the brain stem* is related to the posterior spinal artery and vein, to the posterior medullary segment of the posterior inferior cerebellar artery inferiorly, to the medial posterior choroid artery at its proximal posterior curve and inconstantly to the quadrigeminal portion of the

superior cerebellar artery superiorly. The *cerebellar tonsil* is outlined inferiorly by the tonsillar branch of the posterior inferior cerebellar artery and by the inferior retrotonsillar tributary of the inferior vermian vein. Its antero-medial surface is related to the posterior medullary segment of the posterior inferior cerebellar artery and the retro-olivary vein, its posterior margin is delineated by the retrotonsillar segment of the posterior inferior cerebellar artery and the retro-tonsillar tributaries of the inferior vermian vein so that the antero-posterior dimension of the tonsil can be assessed most easily by the length of the supra-tonsillar segment of the posterior inferior cerebellar artery. This distance also indicates the height of the *4th ventricle*. The upper portion of its roof is indicated by the proximal precentral cerebellar vein and artery the lower portion of the roof by the distal posterior medullary segment of the posterior inferior cerebellar artery. The *vermis* is demarcated anteriorly by the precentral cerebellar vein and artery and the anterior portions of the superior vermian vein and artery, postero-superiorly by the superior vermian vein and artery and inferiorly by the inferior vermian vein and artery. The *cerebello-pontine angle* is assessed by the position of the petrosal vein and the tributaries entering it and by the anterior inferior cerebellar artery with the films taken in straight antero-posterior projection. The *posterior pole of the thalamus* is demarcated by the medial and lateral posterior choroid arteries and the superior thalamic, posterior portion of the internal cerebral and superior choroid veins.

The *splenium of the corpus callosum* is closely related to the splenial artery and vein.

The vessels that are valuable in detecting *midline displacement* in the posterior fossa are the distal posterior medullary segment of the posterior inferior cerebellar artery and its vermian segment and the vermian segment of the superior cerebellar artery. The precentral cerebellar vein may lie to one side proximally but it rarely shows a lateral convexity normally. The inferior vermian vein may be unusually lateral in position but it should not pass across the midline.

It is most important to recognize stretched arteries and veins, whatever their positions, and subtle changes are easily overlooked by the inexperienced.

REFERENCES

[1] Greitz, T. and Löftstedt, S. (1954). 'Relationship between third ventricle and basilar artery.' *Acta Radiol.* **42,** 85–100

[2] Bingas, B. and Cotson, S. (1972). 'Cerebellopontine angle syndrome with uncommon aetiology.' (A case report.) *Neuroradiology* **3,** 165–166

[3] Greitz, T. and Lauren, T. (1968). 'Anterior meningeal branch of the vertebral artery.' *Acta Radiol. (Diag.)* **7,** 219–224

[4] Newton, T. H. (1968). 'The anterior and posterior meningeal branches of the vertebral artery.' *Radiology* **91,** 271–279

[5] Schechter, M. M. and Zingesser, L. H. (1965). 'The anterior spinal artery.' *Acta Radiol. (Diag.)* **3,** 489–496

[6] Stopford, J. B. S. (1916). 'The arteries of the pons and medulla oblongata.' *J. Anat.* **50,** 130–164

[7] Krayenbühl, H. and Yasargil, M. G. (1957). 'Die vaskulären Erkrankungen im Gebiet der Arteria vertebralis und Arteria basialis.' *Fortschr. a.d. Geb. d. Röntgenstrahlen.* Suppl. **80,** 1–170

[8] Takahashi, M., Wilson, G. and Hanafee, W. (1968). 'The anterior inferior cerebellar artery: its radiographic anatomy and significance in the diagnosis of extra-axial tumors of the posterior fossa.' *Radiology* **90,** 281–287

[9] Mani, R. L., Newton, T. H. and Glickman, M. G. (1968). 'The superior cerebellar artery: an anatomic-roentgenographic correlation.' *Radiology* **91,** 1102–1108

[10] Hara, K. and Fujino, Y. (1966). 'The thalamoperforate artery.' *Acta Radiol. (Diag.)* **5,** 192–200

[11] Galloway, J. R. and Greitz, T. (1960). 'The medial and lateral choroid arteries: an anatomic and roentgenographic study.' *Acta Radiol.* **15,** 353–366

[12] Smaltino, F., Bernini, F. P. and Elefante, R. (1971). 'Normal and pathological findings of the angiographic examination of the internal auditory artery.' *Neuroradiology* **2,** 216–222

[13] Margolis, M. T., Newton, T. H. and Hoyt, W. F. (1971). 'Cortical branches of the posterior cerebral artery. Anatomic-radiologic correlation.' *Neuroradiology* **2,** 127–135

[14] Smith, C. G. and Richardson, W. F. (1966). 'The course and distribution of the arteries supplying the visual (striate) cortex.' *Am. J. Ophthal.* **61,** 1391–1396

[15] Huang, Y. P., Wolf, B. S., Antin, S. P. and Okudera, T. (1968). 'The veins of the posterior fossa anterior or petrosal draining group.' *Am. J. Roentgenol.* **104,** 36–56

[16] Gabrielson, T. O. and Amundsen, P. (1969). 'The ponto-mesencephalic veins.' *Radiology* **92,** 889–896

[17] Gabrielson, T. O. and Amundsen, P. (1969). 'The pontine arteries in vertebral angiography.' *Am. J. Roentgenol.* **106,** 296–302

[18] Huang, Y. P., Wolf, B. S., Antin, S. P., Okudera, T. and Kim, I. H. (1968). 'Angiographic features of aqueductal stenosis.' *Am. J. Roentgenol.* **104,** 90–108

[19] Greitz, T. and Sjögren, S. E. (1963). 'The posterior inferior cerebellar artery.' *Acta Radiol. (Diag.)* **1,** 284–297

[20] Krayenbühl, H. and Yasargil, M. G. (1968).

Cerebral Angiography, 2nd edn. London; Butterworths

[21] Takahashi, M., Wilson, G. and Hanafee, W. (1967). The significance of the petrosal vein in the diagnosis of cerebello-pontine angle tumours.' *Radiology* **89**, 834–840

[22] Westberg, G. (1966). 'Arteries of the basal ganglia.' *Acta Radiol. (Diag.)* **5**, 581–596

[23] Bradac, G. B. (1970). 'The ponto-mesencephalic veins.' *Neuroradiology* **1**, 52–57

[24] Huang, Y. P., Wolf, B. S. and Okudera, T. (1969). 'Angiographic anatomy of the inferior vermian vein of the cerebellum.' *Acta Radiol. (Diag.)* **9**, 327–344

[25] Zajgner, J. (1969). 'Normal relationship between basal vein and posterior cerebral artery.' *Acta Radiol. (Diag.)* **9**, 549–552

[26] Giudicelli, G. and Salamon, G. (1970). 'The veins of the thalamus.' *Neuroradiology* **1**, 92–98

[27] Ben Amor, M., Marion, Ch. and Heldt, N. (1971). 'Normal and pathological radio-anatomy of the superior choroid vein.' *Neuroradiology* **3**, 16–19

[28] Serrano, R., Babin, E., Ben Amor, M. and Megret, M. (1972). 'Radio-anatomy of the internal occipital veins.' *Neuroradiology* **3**, 153–154

[29] Huang, Y. P. and Wolf, B. S. (1965). 'The veins of the posterior fossa–superior or galenic draining group.' *Am. J. Roentgenol.* **95**, 808–821

[30] Huang, Y. P. and Wolf, B. S. (1966). 'Pre-central cerebellar vein in angiography.' *Acta Radiol. (Diag.)* **5**, 250–262

[31] Margolis, M. T. and Newton, T. H. (1971). 'An angiographic sign of cerebellar tonsillar herniation.' *Neuroradiology* **2**, 3–8

[32] Wolf, B. S., Newman, C. M. and Khilnani, M. T. (1962). 'The posterior inferior cerebellar artery in vertebral angiography.' *Am. J. Roentgenol.* **87**, 322–337

[33] Billewicz, O. and Heldt, N. (1971). 'The visualisation of the anterior spinal artery and its blood stream direction during brachial vertebral angiography.' *Neuroradiology* **2**, 46–51

[34] Wackenheim, A., Heldt, N. and Ben Amor, M. (1971). 'Variations in the drainage of the lateral mesencephalic vein.' *Neuroradiology* **2**, 154–161

[35] Wolf, B. S., Huang, Y. P. and Newman, C. M. (1963). 'Lateral anastomotic mesencephalic vein and other variations in drainage of the basal cerebral vein.' *Am. J. Roentgenol.* **89**, 411–422

[36] Padget, D. H. (1956). 'Cranial venous system in man in reference to development, adult configuration and relation to arteries.' *Am. J. Anat.* **98**, 307–355

[37] Huang, Y. P. and Wolf, B. S. (1969). 'Angiographic features of fourth ventricle tumors with special reference to the posterior inferior cerebellar artery.' *Am. J. Roentgenol.* **107**, 543–564

[38] Dilenge, D. and David, M. (1967). 'L'angiographie vertebrale.' *Neurochir.* **13**, 121–156

[39] Occleshaw, J. V. (1970). 'The posterior inferior cerebellar arteries. Some quantitative observations in posterior cranial fossa tumours and the Arnold–Chiari malformation.' *Clin. Radiol.* **21**, 1–9

[40] Bories, J., Fredy, D., Rosier, J. and Helias, A. (1970). 'L'angiographie vertebrale. Technique et images normales.' *La Presse Medicale* **78**, 221–224

[41] Johanson, C. (1954). 'Central veins and deep dural sinuses of the brain: an anatomical and angiographic study.' *Acta Radiol.* Suppl. 107, 1–184

[42] Stephens, R. B. and Stilwell, D. L. (1969). *Arteries and Veins of the Human Brain*. Springfield, Illinois; Thomas

[43] Ben Amor, M. and Billewicz, O. (1970). 'The posterior cerebral vein.' *Neuroradiology* **1**, 179–182

[44] Wackenheim, A. and Braun, J. P. (1970). *Angiography of the Mesencephalon*. Berlin; Springer

[45] Bull, J. W. D. and Kozlowski, P. (1970). 'The angiographic pattern of the petrosal veins in the normal and pathological.' *Neuroradiology* **1**, 20–26

[46] Ross, F., du Boulay, G. H. and Keller, B. (1975). 'Normal measurements in angiography of the posterior fossa.' *Radiology* **116**, 335–340

[47] Huang, Y. P. and Wolf, B. S. (1967). 'The vein of the lateral recess of the fourth ventricle and its tributaries. Roentgen appearance and anatomic relationships.' *Am. J. Roentgenol.* **101**, 1–21

[48] Belloni, G. and du Boulay, G. H. (1974). 'The choroidal point and the copular point.' *Br. J. Radiol.* **47**, 261–264

NOTES ABOUT THE ILLUSTRATIONS

In the drawings, perspective and contrast have been used to indicate what is near, what is far, and what is seen through brain substance. The smaller branches and tributaries have been omitted. Naturally, only one of the infinite number of variations of detailed anatomy has been illustrated in each of these pictures.

In the diagrammatic representations of the copular, choroidal and colliculo-central points we have followed the references given in our text. We would like to add that while this book was in production, Belloni and du Boulay reviewed a large material and formulated the idea of using the actual origin of the choroidal branch of the posterior inferior cerebellar artery as the choroidal point. It can be seen in the lateral view in 80 per cent of cases. Belloni's choroidal point lies, on average, slightly posterior to that defined by Huang and Wolf[37]. Belloni and du Boulay[48] also give new measurements for the position of the copular point. Ross and du Boulay have made a detailed quantitative study of the position of many of the vessels in the posterior cranial fossa.

The subtraction radiographs have been arranged so that a lateral view is always available on the open page for comparison with the Towne's or antero-posterior view. This has dictated the repetition of a few of the laterals.

Heavy black diagrammatic lines mark the clivus, the petrous ridges or the inner table of the occipital and parietal bones. In the lateral views the line is drawn on the midline profile of the occipital bone and therefore the vessels of the dorsal parts of the cerebellar hemisphere sometimes bulge beyond it.

In some places a suffix has been employed to distinguish one side from the other when paired arteries have both been numbered, thus 7 and 7′.

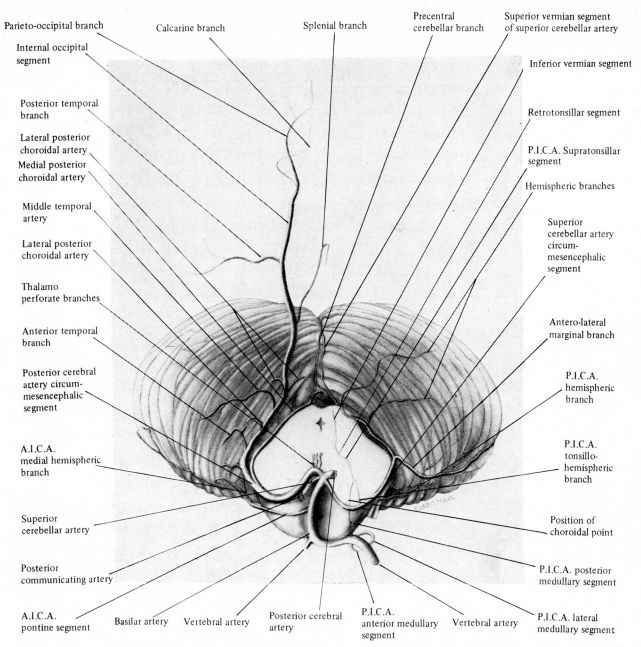

Parieto-occipital branch

Internal occipital segment

Posterior temporal branch

Lateral posterior choroidal artery

Medial posterior choroidal artery

Middle temporal artery

Lateral posterior choroidal artery

Thalamo perforate branches

Anterior temporal branch

Posterior cerebral artery circum-mesencephalic segment

A.I.C.A. medial hemispheric branch

Superior cerebellar artery

Posterior communicating artery

A.I.C.A. pontine segment

Calcarine branch

Basilar artery

Vertebral artery

Splenial branch

Posterior cerebral artery

Precentral cerebellar branch

P.I.C.A. anterior medullary segment

Superior vermian segment of superior cerebellar artery

Inferior vermian segment

Retrotonsillar segment

P.I.C.A. Supratonsillar segment

Hemispheric branches

Superior cerebellar artery circum-mesencephalic segment

Antero-lateral marginal branch

P.I.C.A. hemispheric branch

P.I.C.A. tonsillo-hemispheric branch

Position of choroidal point

Vertebral artery

P.I.C.A. posterior medullary segment

P.I.C.A. lateral medullary segment

Figure 1—The cerebellum, midbrain and pons seen from in front and above. The tentorium has been removed, as well as the cerebrum, and the posterior cerebral artery is lying free in space. Note that almost all of the posterior inferior cerebellar artery is seen through the brain stem and cerebellum.

19

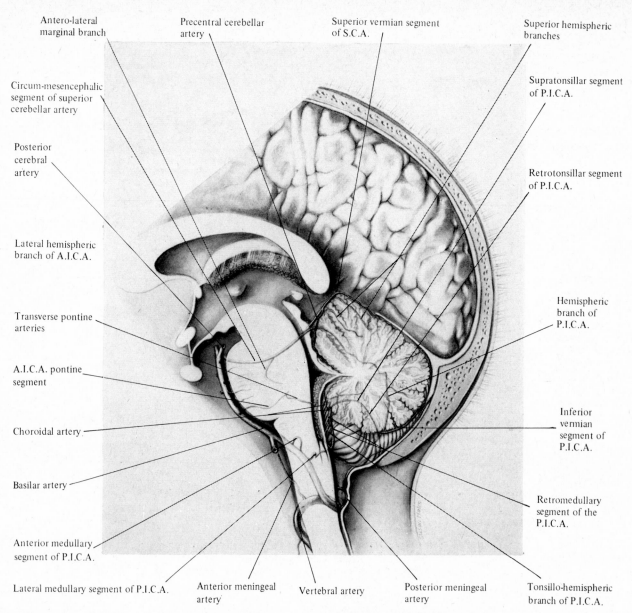

Antero-lateral marginal branch

Precentral cerebellar artery

Superior vermian segment of S.C.A.

Superior hemispheric branches

Circum-mesencephalic segment of superior cerebellar artery

Posterior cerebral artery

Lateral hemispheric branch of A.I.C.A.

Transverse pontine arteries

A.I.C.A. pontine segment

Choroidal artery

Basilar artery

Anterior medullary segment of P.I.C.A.

Supratonsillar segment of P.I.C.A.

Retrotonsillar segment of P.I.C.A.

Hemispheric branch of P.I.C.A.

Inferior vermian segment of P.I.C.A.

Retromedullary segment of the P.I.C.A.

Tonsillo-hemispheric branch of P.I.C.A.

Lateral medullary segment of P.I.C.A.

Anterior meningeal artery

Vertebral artery

Posterior meningeal artery

Figure 2—Lateral view after sagittal section and removal of the falx. Note that most of the arteries shown are on the far side. The posterior cerebrals have been cut away to show the superior cerebellar artery more clearly.

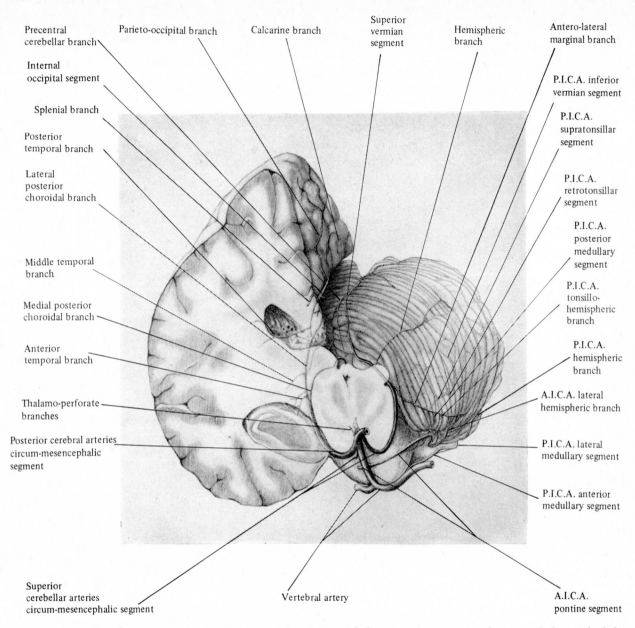

Precentral cerebellar branch

Internal occipital segment

Splenial branch

Posterior temporal branch

Lateral posterior choroidal branch

Middle temporal branch

Medial posterior choroidal branch

Anterior temporal branch

Thalamo-perforate branches

Posterior cerebral arteries circum-mesencephalic segment

Superior cerebellar arteries circum-mesencephalic segment

Parieto-occipital branch

Calcarine branch

Superior vermian segment

Hemispheric branch

Antero-lateral marginal branch

P.I.C.A. inferior vermian segment

P.I.C.A. supratonsillar segment

P.I.C.A. retrotonsillar segment

P.I.C.A. posterior medullary segment

P.I.C.A. tonsillo-hemispheric branch

P.I.C.A. hemispheric branch

A.I.C.A. lateral hemispheric branch

P.I.C.A. lateral medullary segment

P.I.C.A. anterior medullary segment

Vertebral artery

A.I.C.A. pontine segment

Figure 3—Oblique anterior view. A coronal section has been made but not quite square to the sagittal plane. The left cerebral hemisphere has thus been completely removed, but not the right.

21

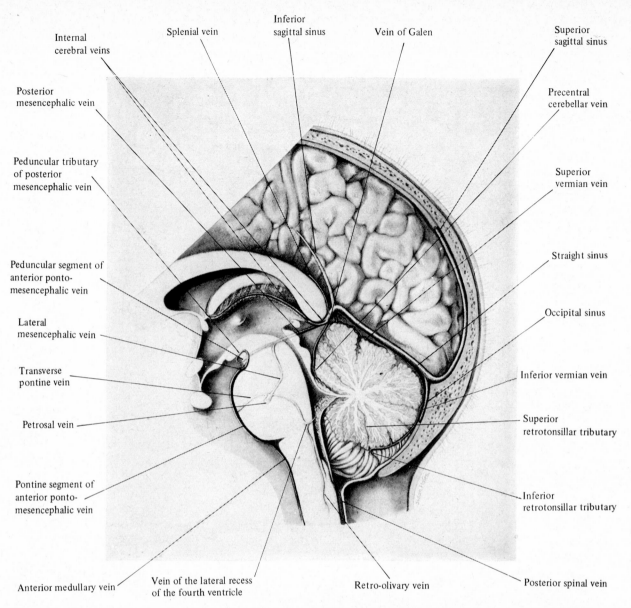

Internal
cerebral veins

Splenial vein

Inferior
sagittal sinus

Vein of Galen

Superior
sagittal sinus

Posterior
mesencephalic vein

Precentral
cerebellar vein

Peduncular tributary
of posterior
mesencephalic vein

Superior
vermian vein

Peduncular segment of
anterior ponto-
mesencephalic vein

Straight sinus

Lateral
mesencephalic vein

Occipital sinus

Transverse
pontine vein

Inferior vermian vein

Petrosal vein

Superior
retrotonsillar tributary

Pontine segment of
anterior ponto-
mesencephalic vein

Inferior
retrotonsillar tributary

Anterior medullary vein

Vein of the lateral recess
of the fourth ventricle

Retro-olivary vein

Posterior spinal vein

Figure 4—Lateral view after sagittal section. Note that the faintly shaded veins are on the other side of the brain stem. The falx and tentorium have not been represented.

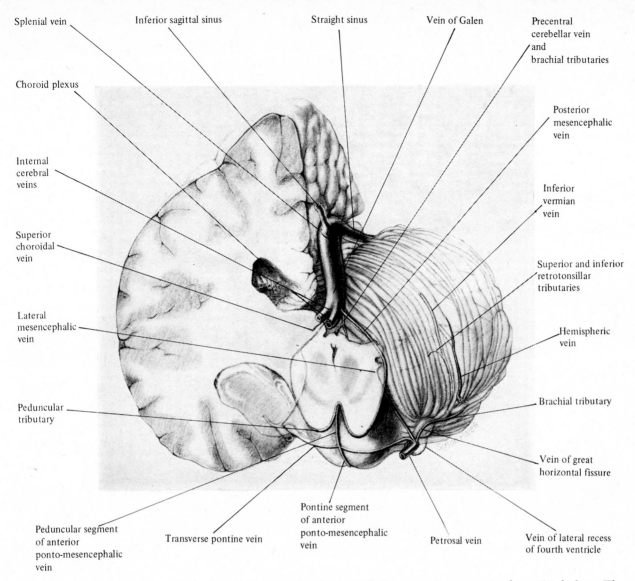

Splenial vein

Inferior sagittal sinus

Straight sinus

Vein of Galen

Precentral
cerebellar vein
and
brachial tributaries

Choroid plexus

Posterior
mesencephalic
vein

Internal
cerebral
veins

Inferior
vermian
vein

Superior
choroidal
vein

Superior and inferior
retrotonsillar
tributaries

Lateral
mesencephalic
vein

Hemispheric
vein

Peduncular
tributary

Brachial tributary

Vein of great
horizontal fissure

Peduncular segment
of anterior
ponto-mesencephalic
vein

Transverse pontine vein

Pontine segment
of anterior
ponto-mesencephalic
vein

Petrosal vein

Vein of lateral recess
of fourth ventricle

Figure 5—Oblique anterior view. A coronal section has been made but not quite square to the sagittal plane. The left cerebral hemisphere has thus been completely removed, but not the right. The tentorium is not represented.

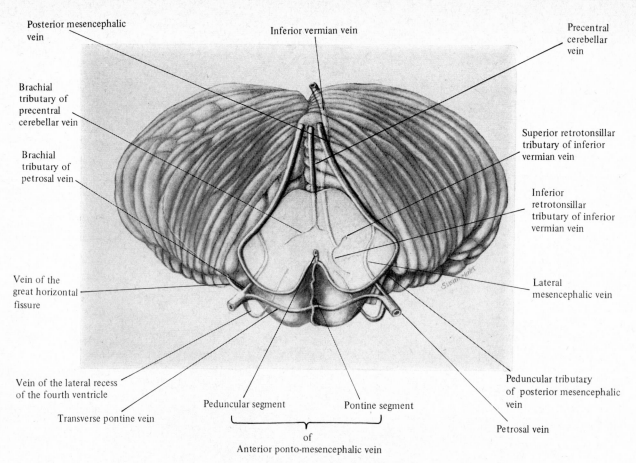

Posterior mesencephalic vein

Inferior vermian vein

Precentral cerebellar vein

Brachial tributary of precentral cerebellar vein

Brachial tributary of petrosal vein

Superior retrotonsillar tributary of inferior vermian vein

Inferior retrotonsillar tributary of inferior vermian vein

Vein of the great horizontal fissure

Lateral mesencephalic vein

Vein of the lateral recess of the fourth ventricle

Peduncular tributary of posterior mesencephalic vein

Transverse pontine vein

Peduncular segment

Pontine segment

Petrosal vein

of
Anterior ponto-mesencephalic vein

Figure 6—The cerebellum, midbrain and pons seen from in front and above.

24

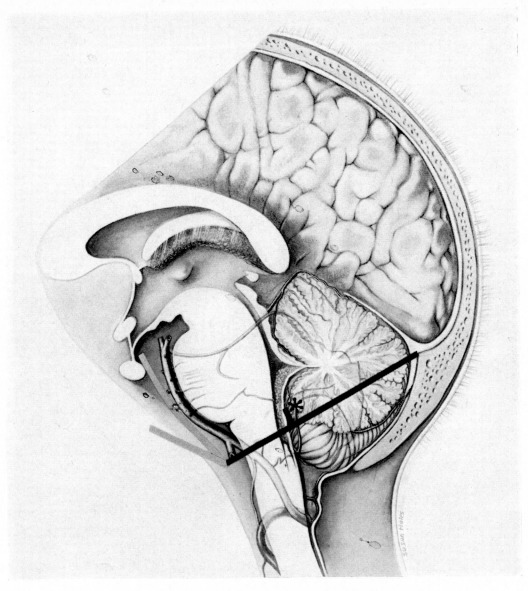

Figure 7—The choroidal point.

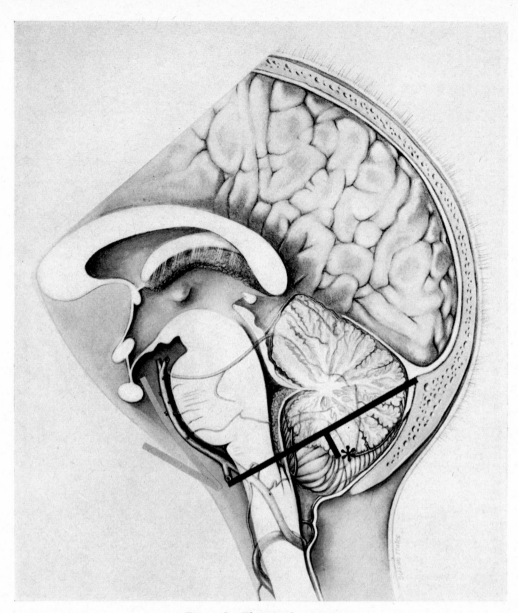

Figure 8—The copular point.

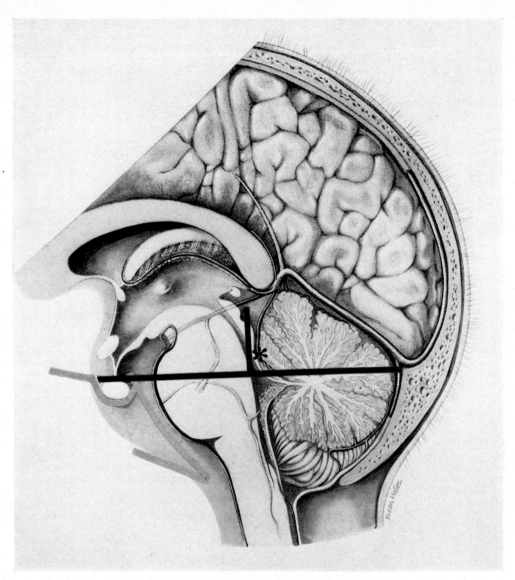

Figure 9—The colliculo-central point.

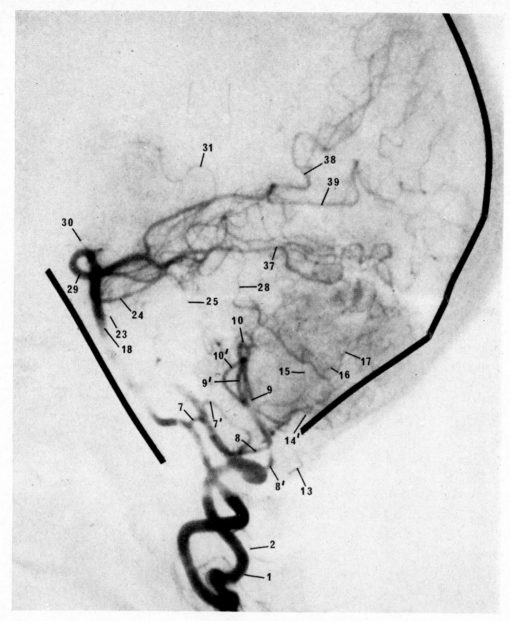

Figure 10

Case 1 (Figures 10–13)—Arterial system. Lateral, Towne's and antero-posterior views. Both posterior inferior cerebellar arteries are filled and separately labelled. Note that the two choroidal points lie at different levels. Only one posterior cerebral artery has been outlined and this makes it easy to understand in the lateral view.

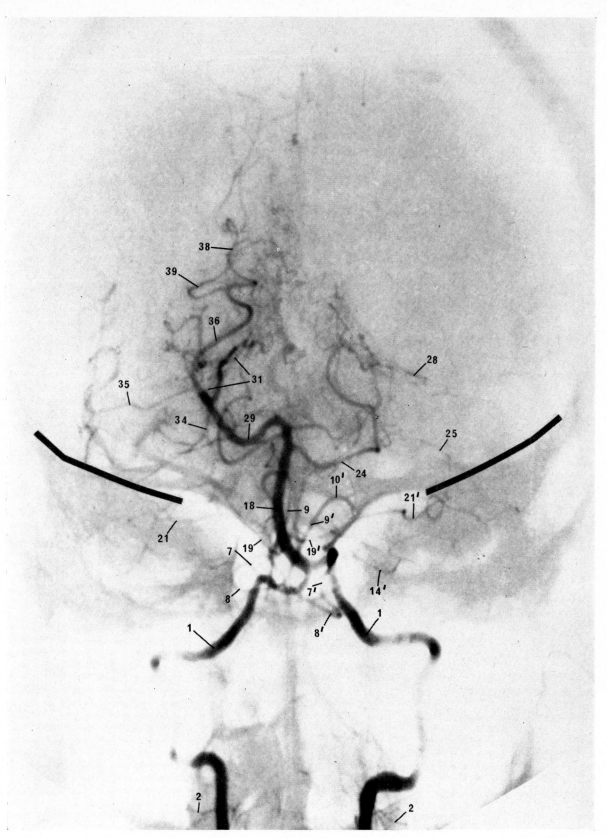

Figure 11

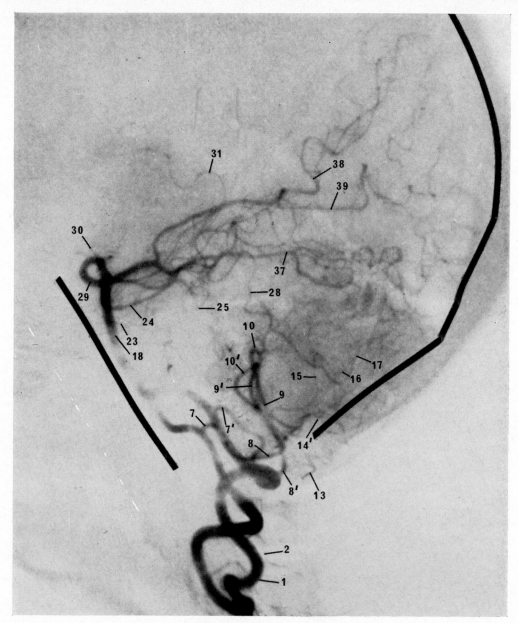

Figure 12

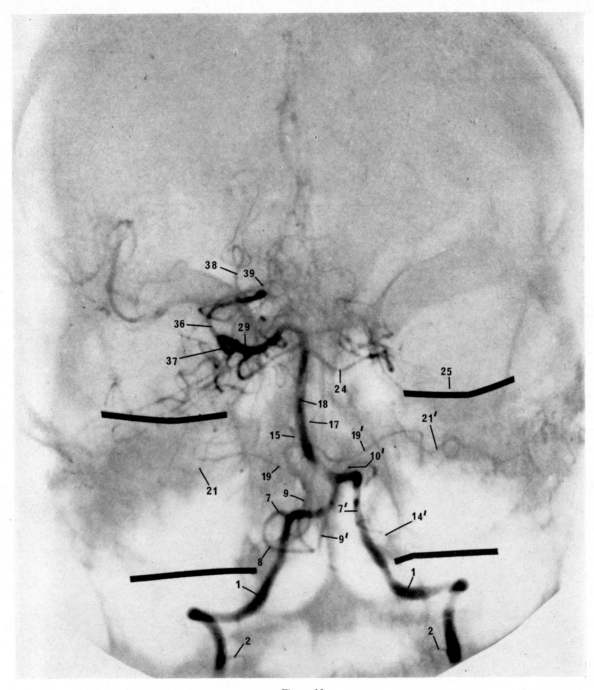

Figure 13

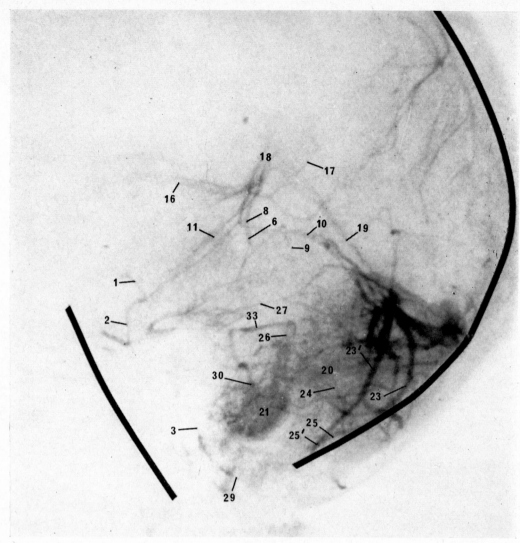

Figure 14

Case 1 (Figures 14 and 15)—Venous systems. Lateral and Towne's views. The two inferior vermian veins are asymmetrical. One lies on the vermis itself, and the other, a little further from the midline, crosses the medial surface of the cerebellar hemisphere. The lateral mesencephalic veins are poorly developed.

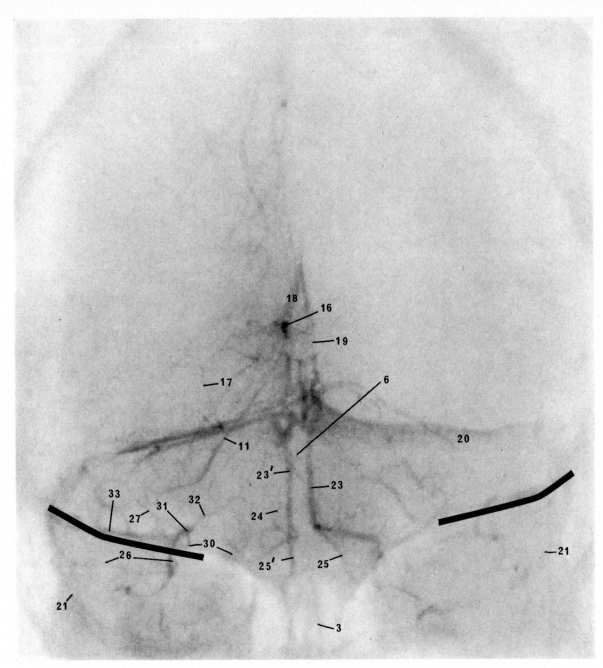

Figure 15

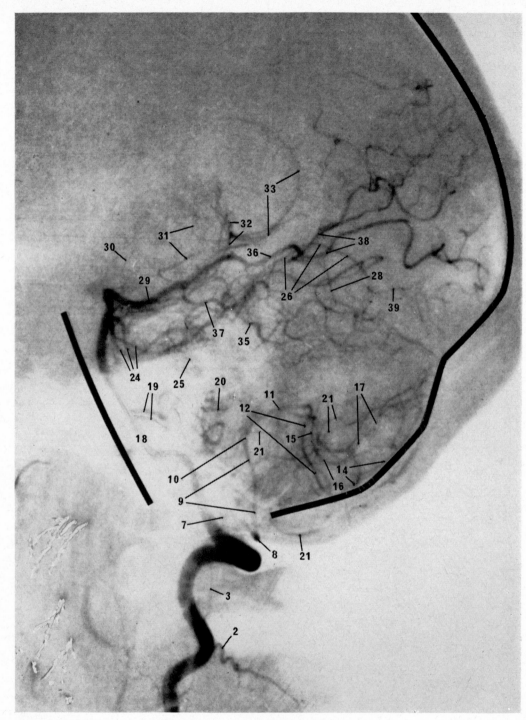

Figure 16

Case 2 (Figures 16 and 17)—Arterial system. Lateral and Towne's views. Only one posterior cerebral artery is filled, so the branches are easy to distinguish in the lateral view. The anterior inferior cerebellar arteries are exceptionally large and important.

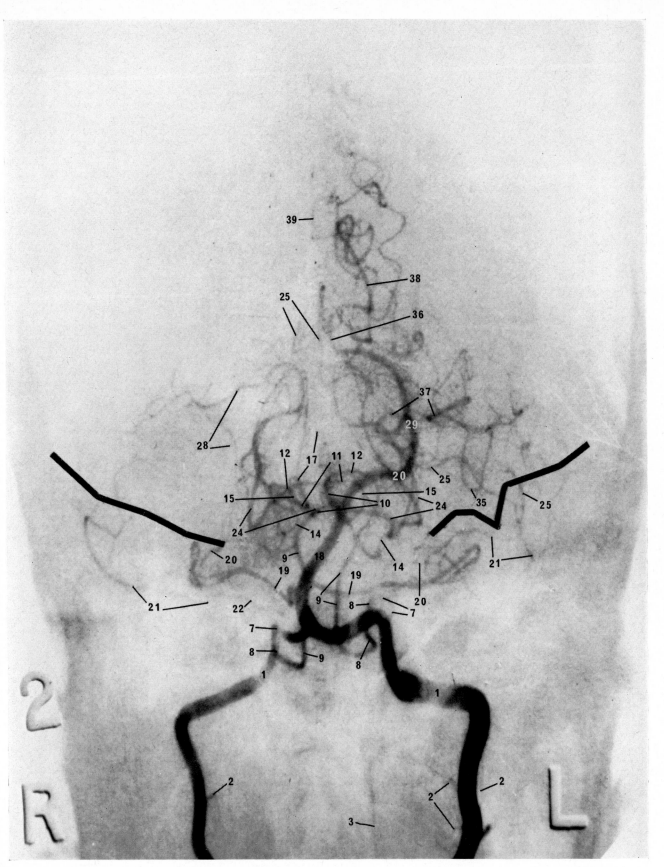

Figure 17

35

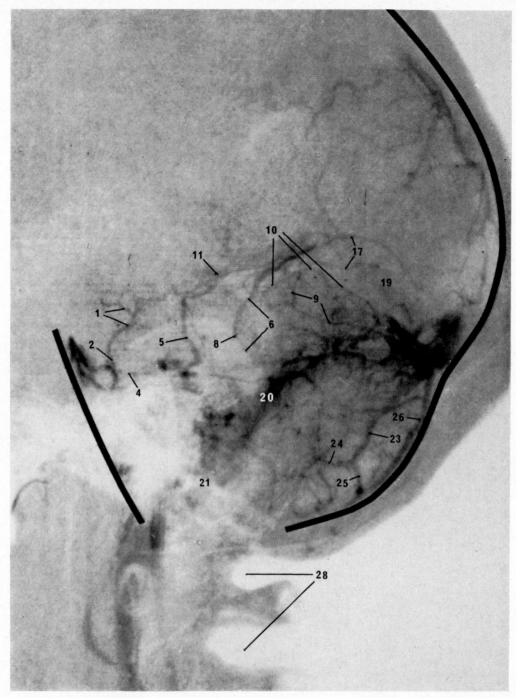

Figure 18

Case 2 (*Figures 18 and 19*)—*Venous system. Lateral and Towne's views. The pre-central cerebellar vein is superimposed upon one inferior vermian vein in the Towne's view, but can be recognized by its brachial tributaries.*

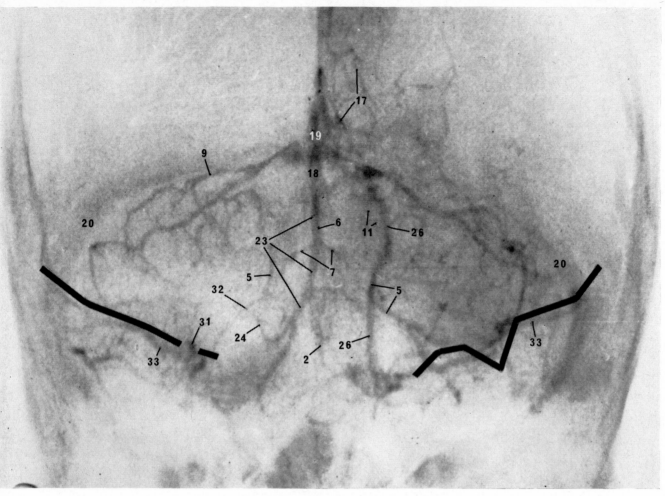

Figure 19

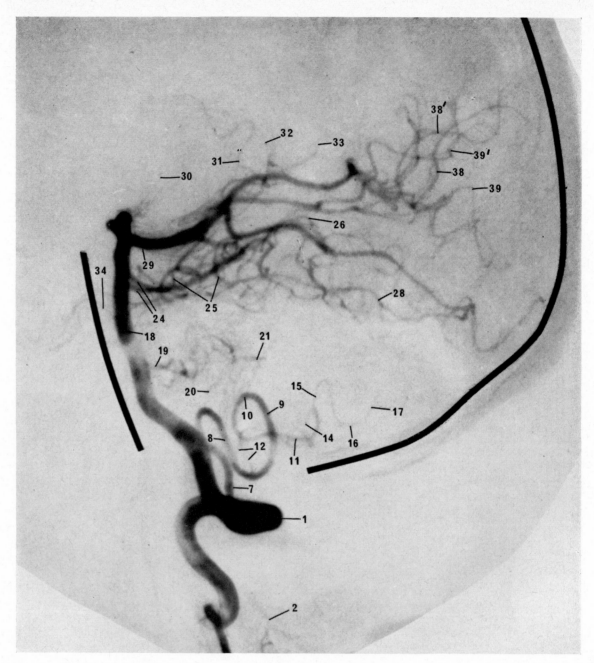

Figure 20

Case 3 (Figures 20 and 21)—*Arterial system. Lateral and Towne's views. Both posterior cerebral arteries are filled, but it is possible to distinguish their branches in the lateral view. The anterior inferior cerebellar artery and left posterior inferior cerebellar artery are large arteries. The two terminal branches of the anterior inferior cerebellar artery are both identifiable. The segment of the posterior inferior cerebellar artery which courses over the medial surface of the tonsil cannot be called 'supratonsillar' because of its relatively inferior position. The best available name is 'medial tonsillar segment'.*

38

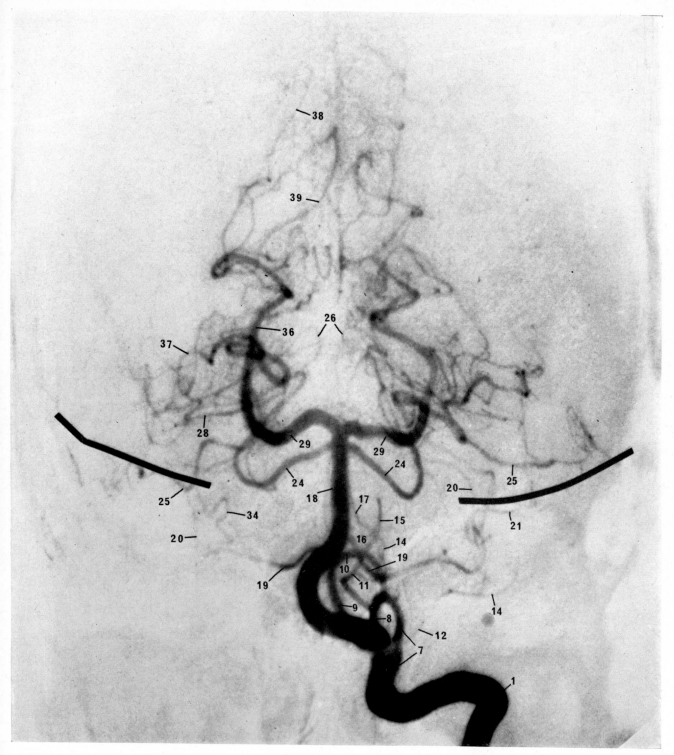

Figure 21

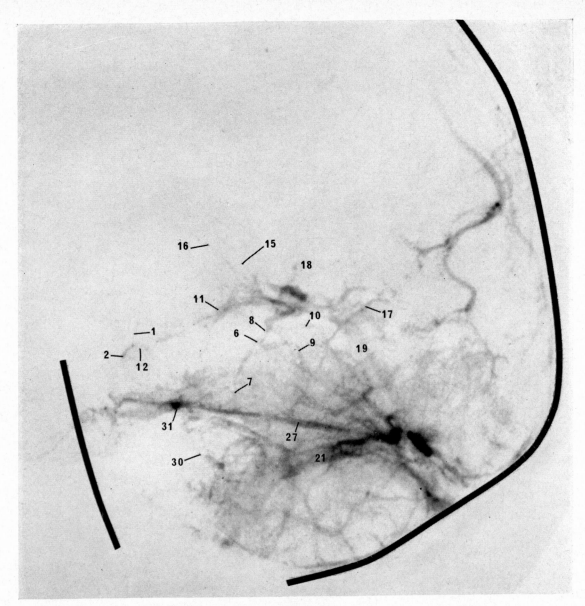

Figure 22

Case 3 (Figures 22 and 23)—Venous system. Lateral and Towne's views. Note the anastomosis in this case between the brachial tributaries of the pre-central cerebellar vein and the lateral mesencephalic vein.

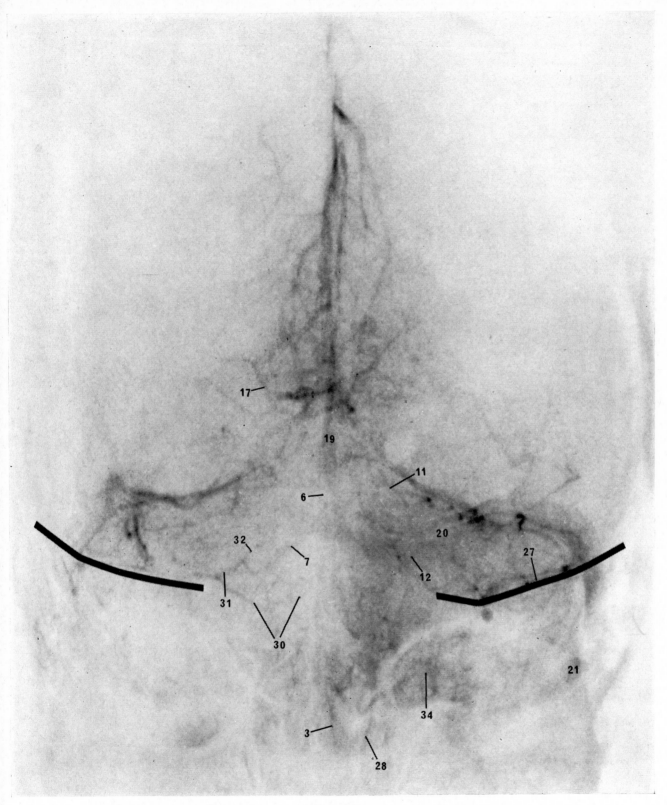

Figure 23

41

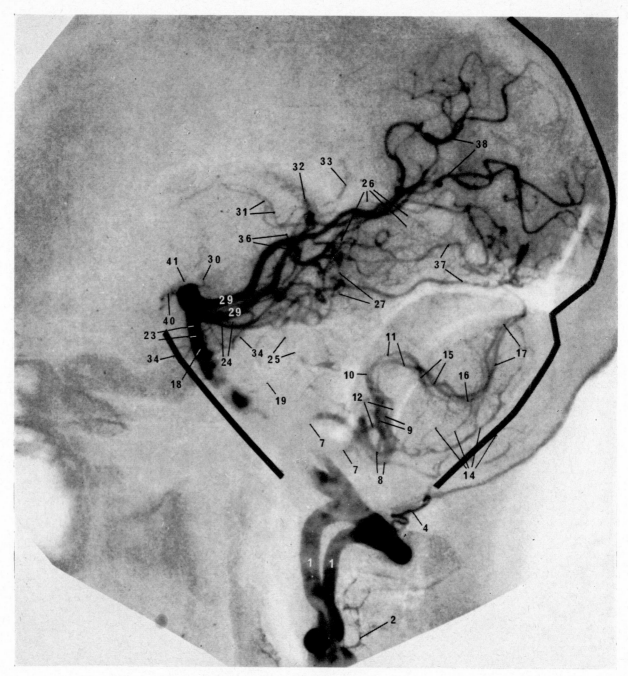

Figure 24

Case 4 (Figures 24–27)—*Arterial system. Lateral, Towne's and antero-posterior views. The two posterior inferior cerebellar arteries are remarkably symmetrical. The value of the antero-posterior view for the anterior inferior cerebellar artery and the hemispheric branches of the posterior inferior cerebellar artery is obvious. The posterior meningeal artery is visible.*

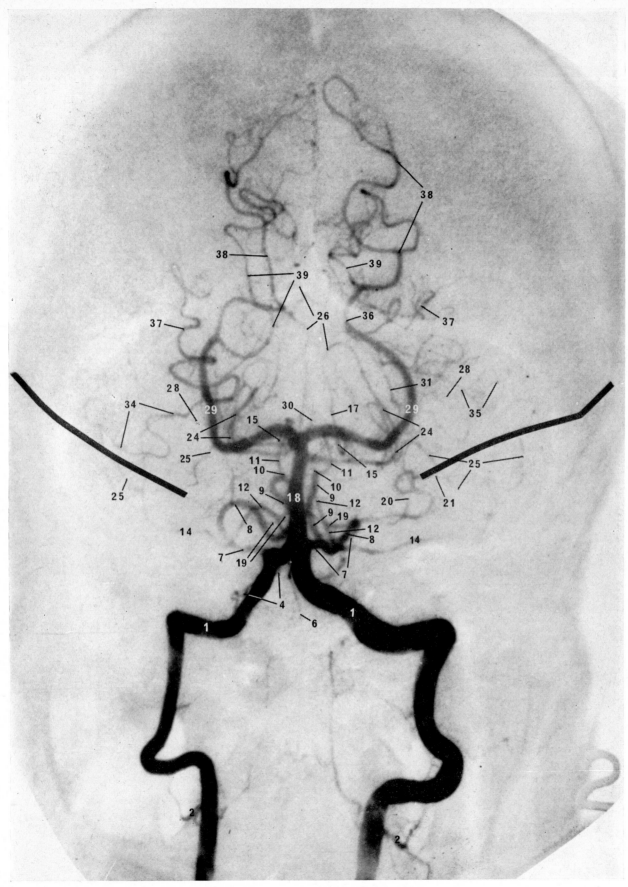

Figure 25

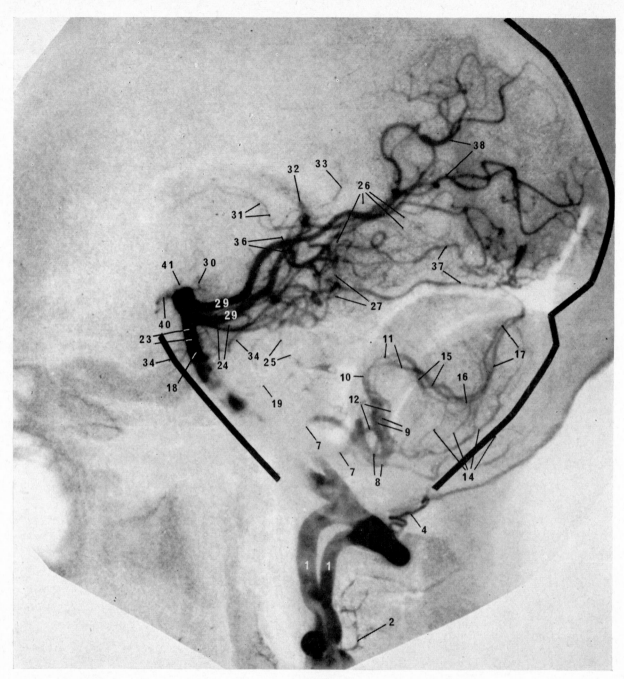

Figure 26

44

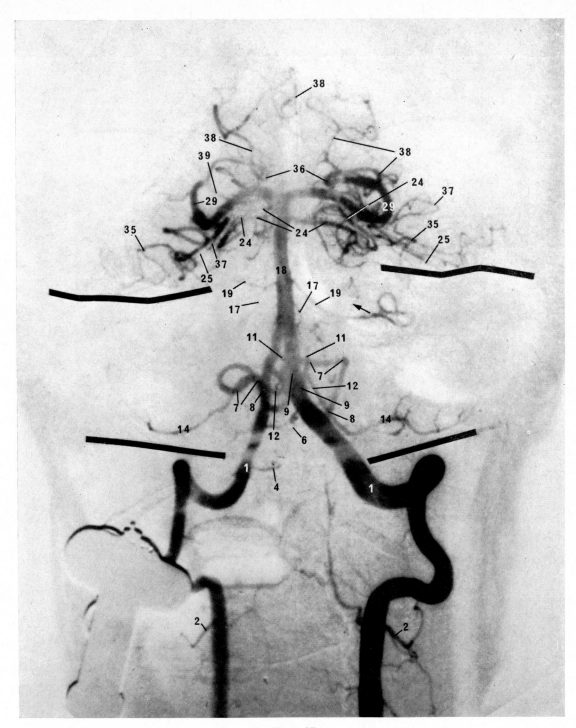

Figure 27

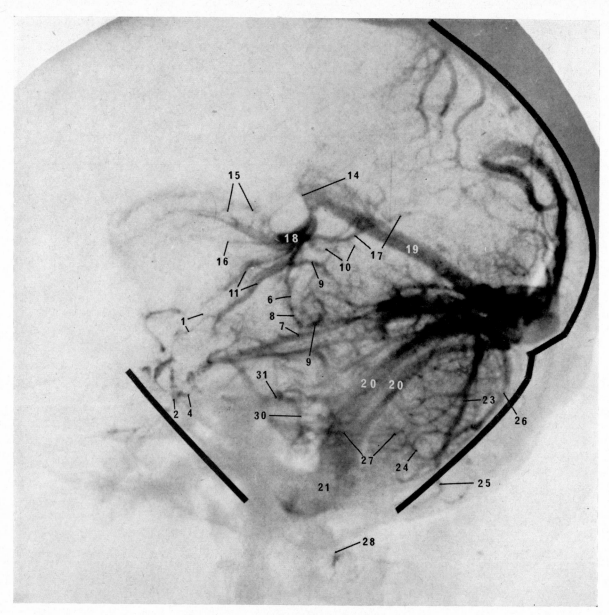

Figure 28

Case 4 (*Figures 28 and 29*)—*Venous system. Lateral and Towne's views. The lateral view shows the posterior spinal vein.*

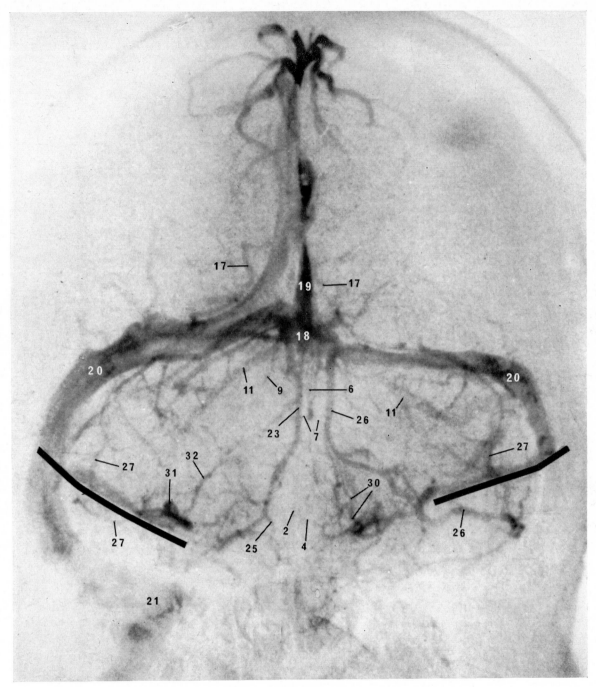

Figure 29

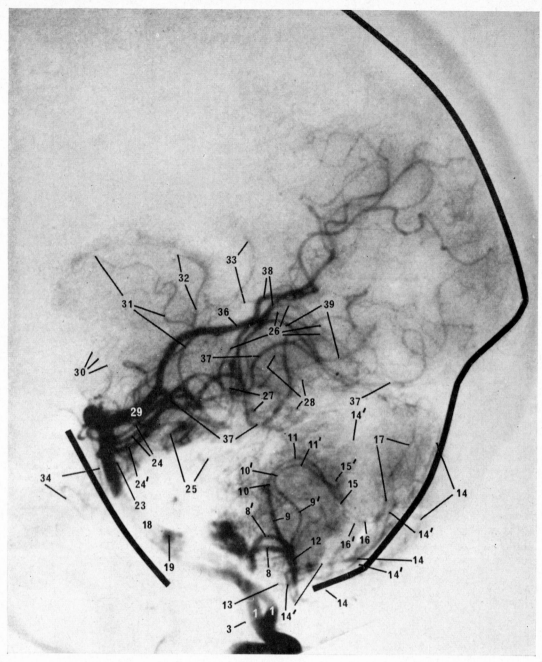

Figure 30

Case 5 (Figures 30 and 31)—Arterial system. Lateral and Towne's views. An anterior temporal branch of the posterior cerebral artery is clearly shown. Terminal branches of both the superior and posterior inferior cerebellar arteries reveal a convincingly symmetrical disposition on either side of the midline. Note in the lateral view that the vasculature of the cerebellar hemispheres juts out beyond the black line marking the inner table of the vault in the midline.

48

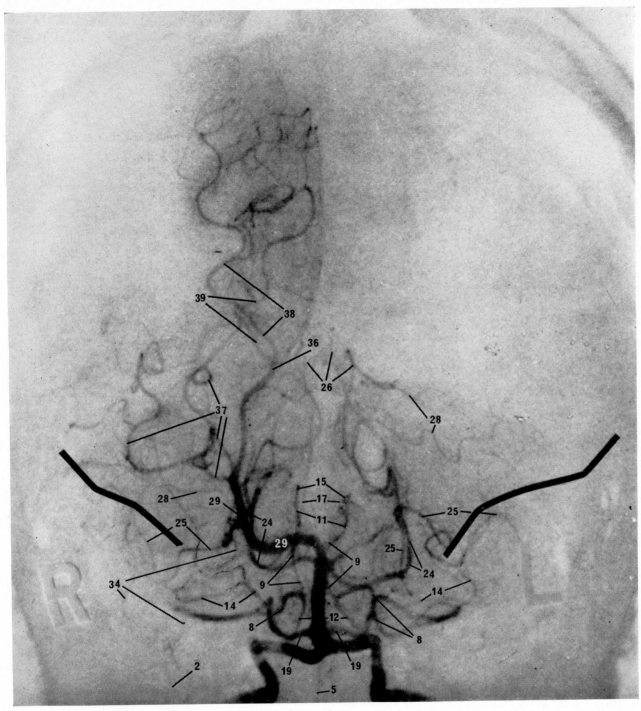

Figure 31

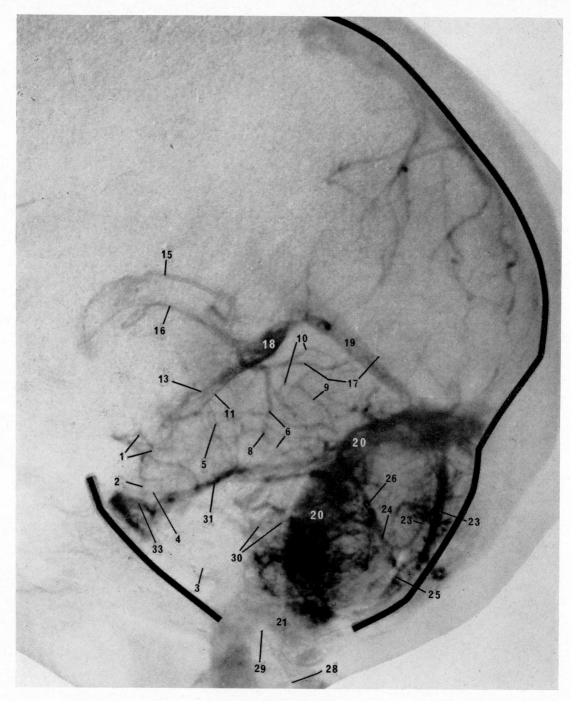

Figure 32

Case 5 (Figures 32 and 33)—Venous system. Lateral and Towne's views. The lateral mesencephalic veins are especially well shown.

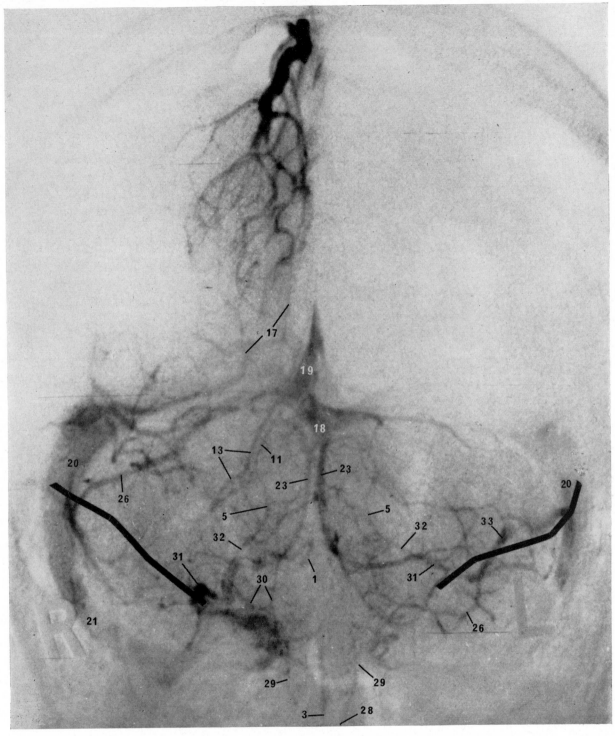

Figure 33

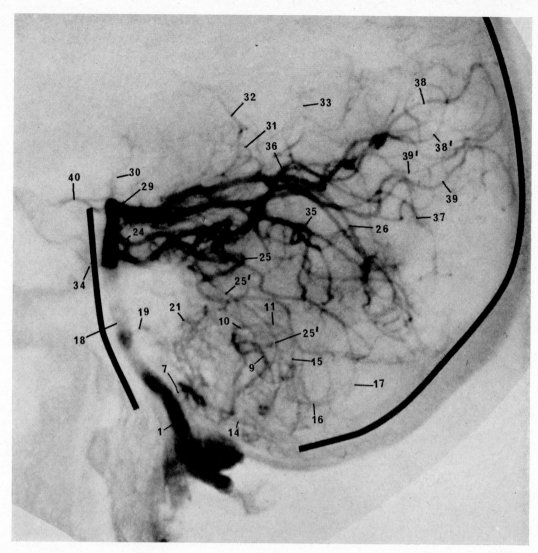

Figure 34

Case 6 (Figures 34 and 35)—Arterial system. Lateral and Towne's views. There is an exceptionally large antero-lateral marginal branch of the right superior cerebellar artery.

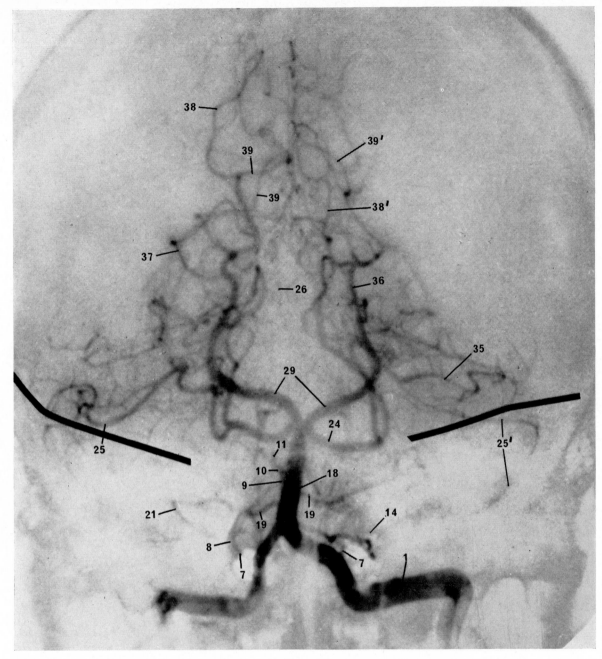

Figure 35

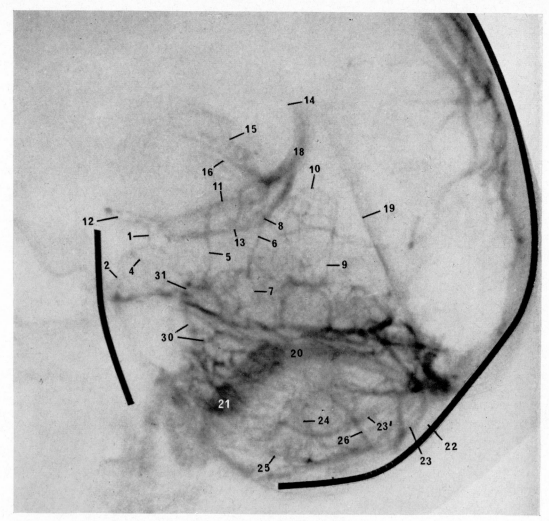

Figure 36

Case 6 (Figures 36 and 37)—Venous system. Lateral and Towne's views. On one side the basal vein of Rosenthal has been filled, on the other the posterior mesencephalic.

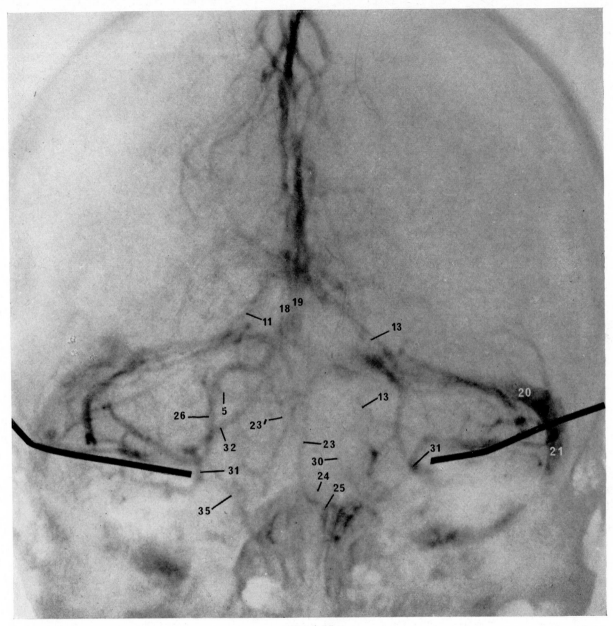

Figure 37

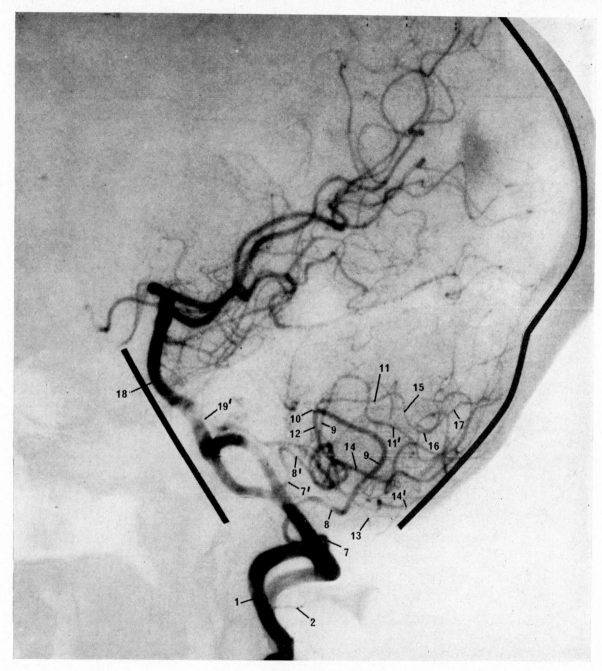

Figure 38

Case 7 (Figures 38 and 39)—Arterial system. Lateral and Towne's views. There is exceptionally good filling of both posterior inferior cerebellar arteries. Note what a bad guide the posterior medullary segment is to the position of the posterior surface of the brain stem.

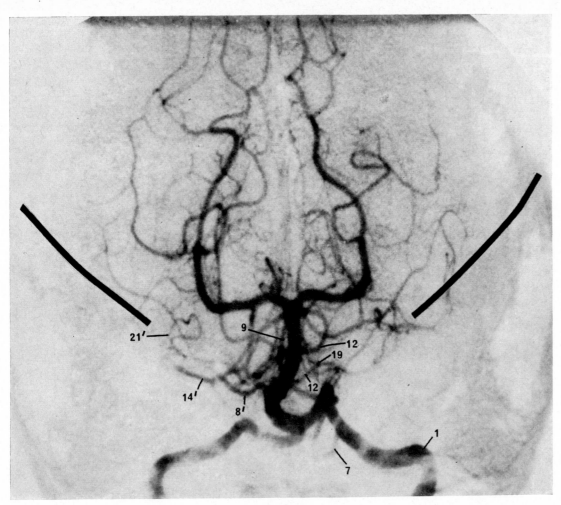

Figure 39

57

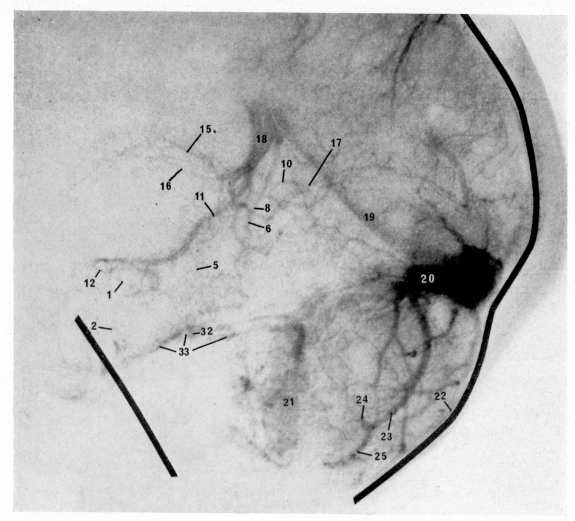

Figure 40

Case 7 (Figures 40 and 41)—*Venous system. Lateral and Towne's views. One of the few cases in which the occipital sinus is visible. Transverse pontine veins are also very nicely shown and the superior petrosal sinuses are large.*

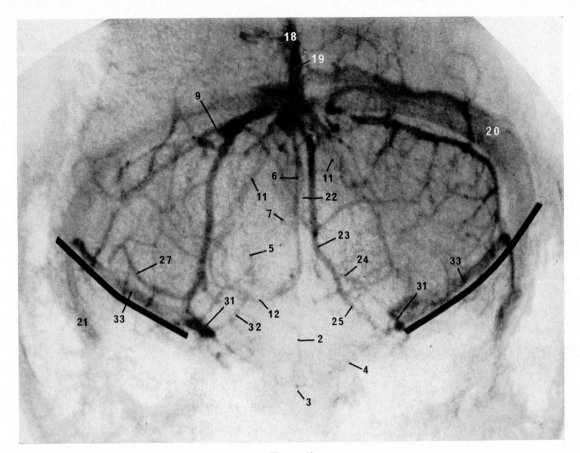

Figure 41

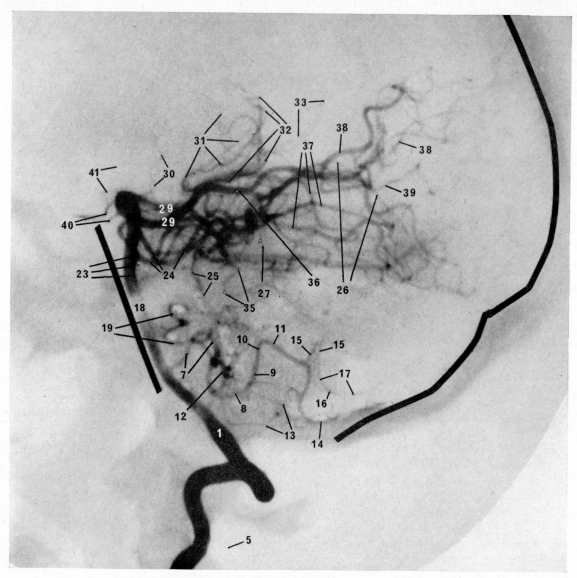

Figure 42

Case 8 (Figures 42 and 43)—*Arterial system. Lateral and Towne's views. This is one of the examples in which the medial posterior choroidal artery can be seen in the Towne's view.*

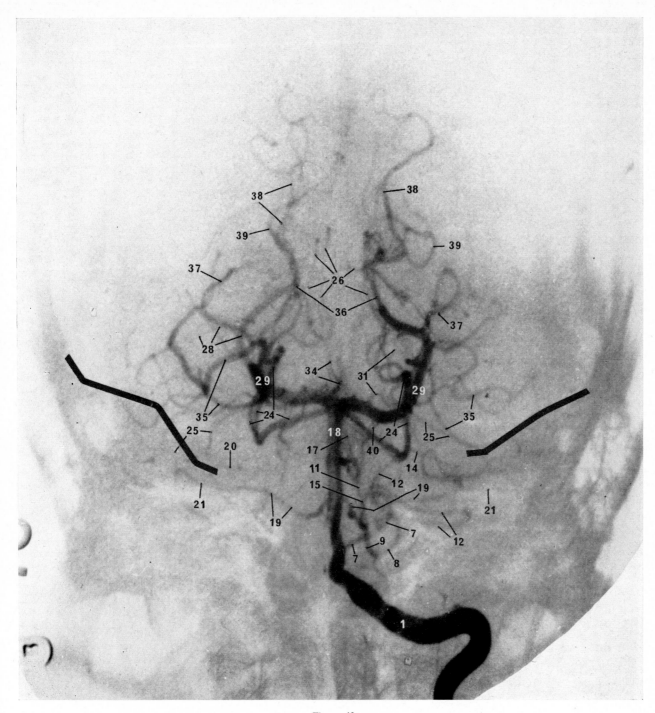

Figure 43

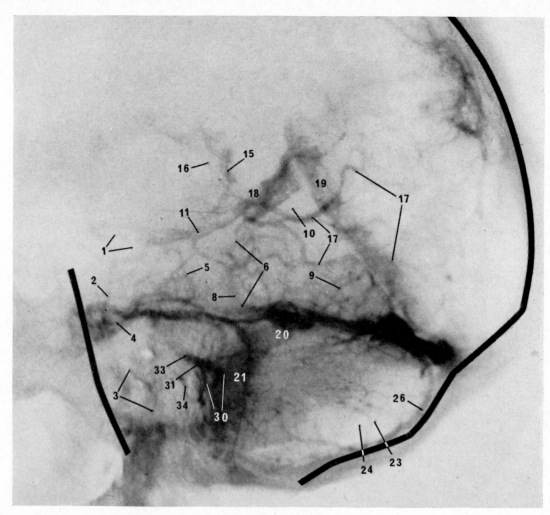

Figure 44

Case 8 (*Figures 44 and 45*)—*Venous system. Lateral and Towne's views. An anterior medullary vein can just be made out.*

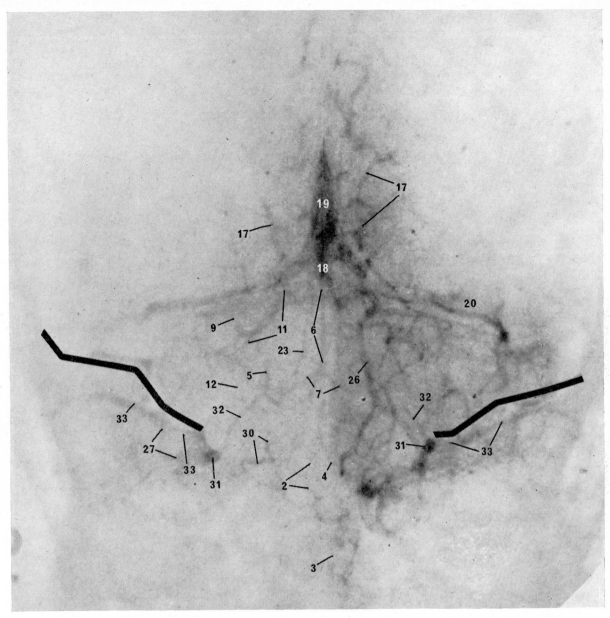

Figure 45

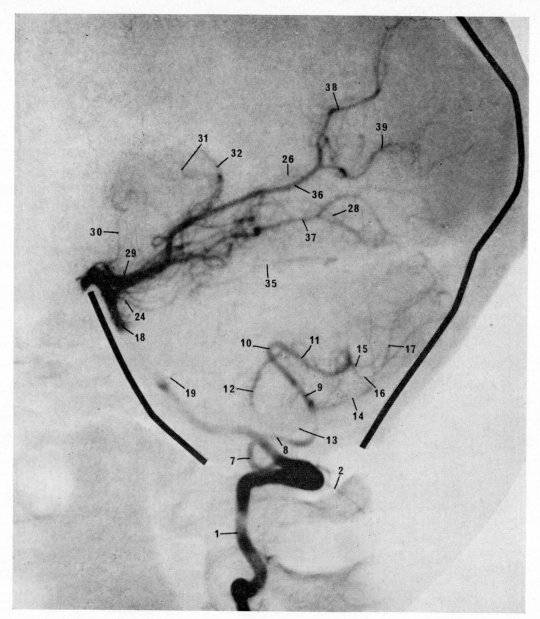

Figure 46

Case 9 (*Figures 46 and 47*)—*Arterial system. Lateral and Towne's views. The posterior inferior cerebellar artery exhibits a typical anatomical course as described in most standard works. One of the thalamo-perforate arteries is large and especially easy to see.*

64

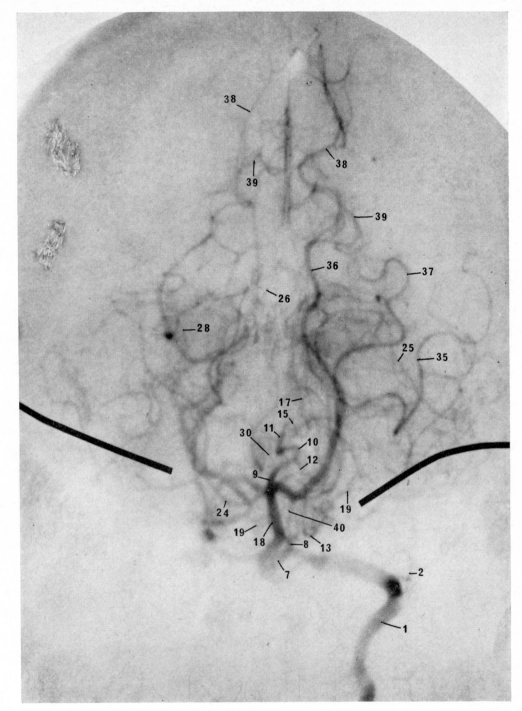

Figure 47

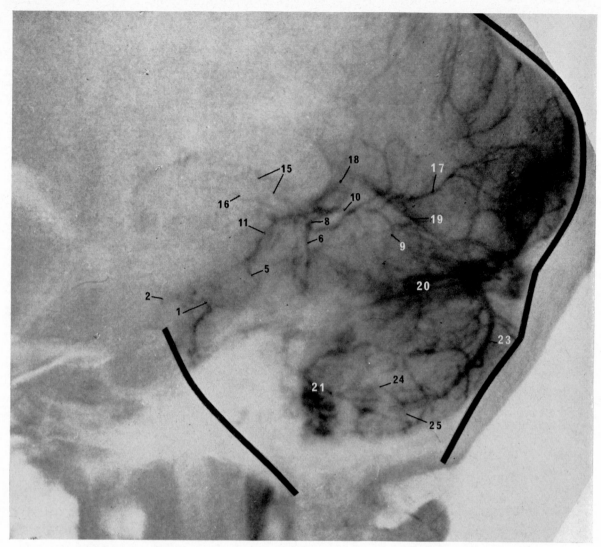

Figure 48

Case 9 (Figures 48 and 49)—Venous system. Lateral and Towne's views. Note the anterior ponto-mesencephalic vein.

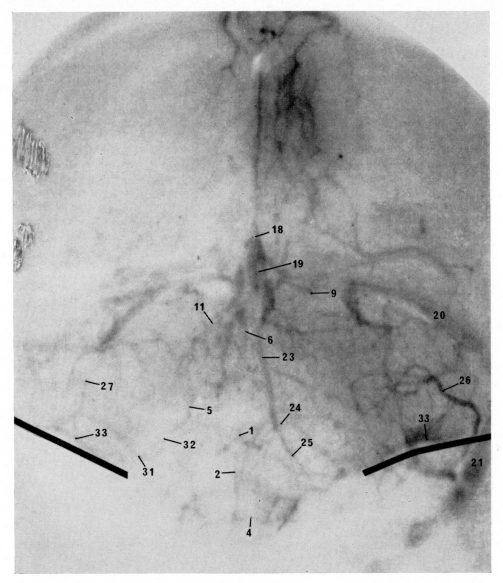

Figure 49

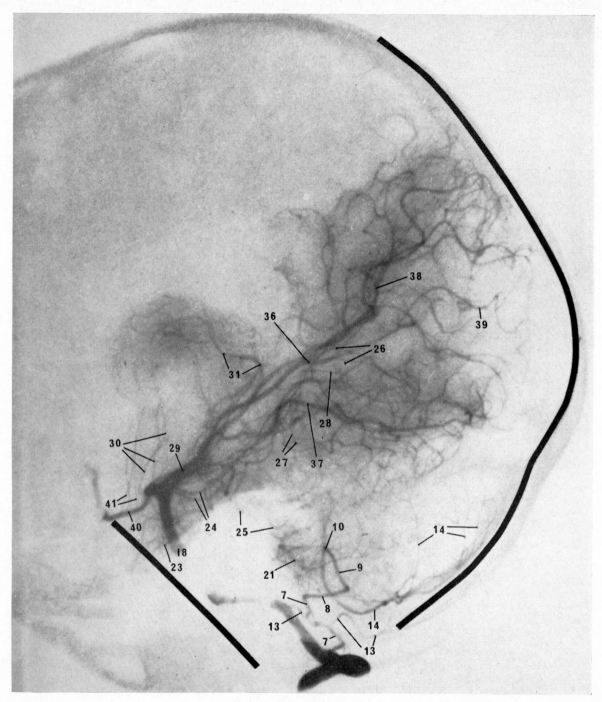

Figure 50

Case 10 (Figures 50 and 51) Arterial system. Lateral and Towne's views. The posterior inferior cerebellar artery has no supra-tonsillar segment, but its function is served by a hemispheric branch. The tonsillar branch is separate. Note the very large medial posterior choroidal arteries.

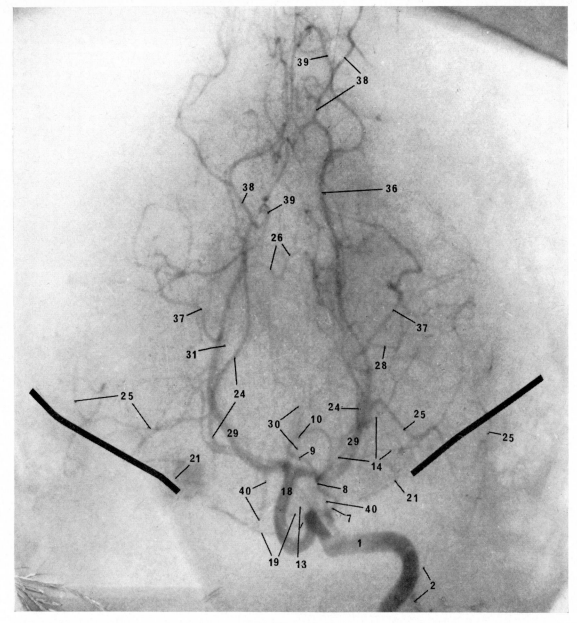

Figure 51

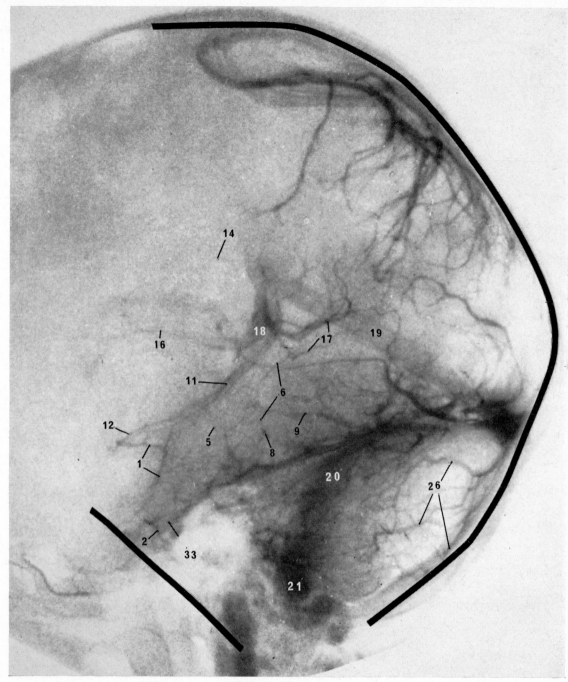

Figure 52

Case 10 (Figures 52 and 53)—Venous system. Lateral and Towne's views. The Towne's view gives a helpful picture of both the vein of the lateral recess of the 4th ventricle and the peduncular tributary of the posterior mesencephalic vein.

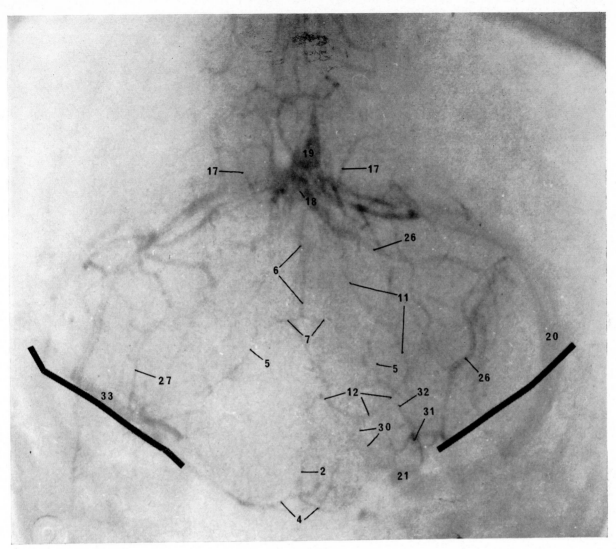

Figure 53

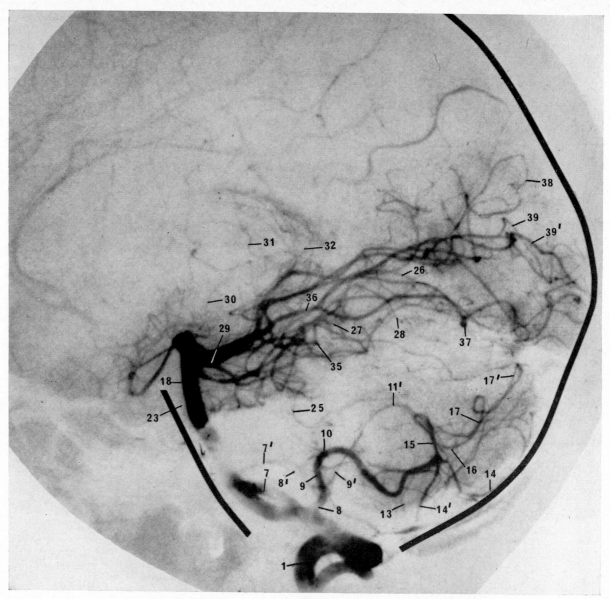

Figure 54

Case 11 (Figures 54–57)—*Arterial system. Lateral, Towne's and antero-posterior views. Note that both posterior inferior cerebellar arteries are filled, the left one being much the larger, and that their relationships with the two tonsils are different. On the right there is a supratonsillar segment; on the left the corresponding portion of the artery lies at a much lower level.*

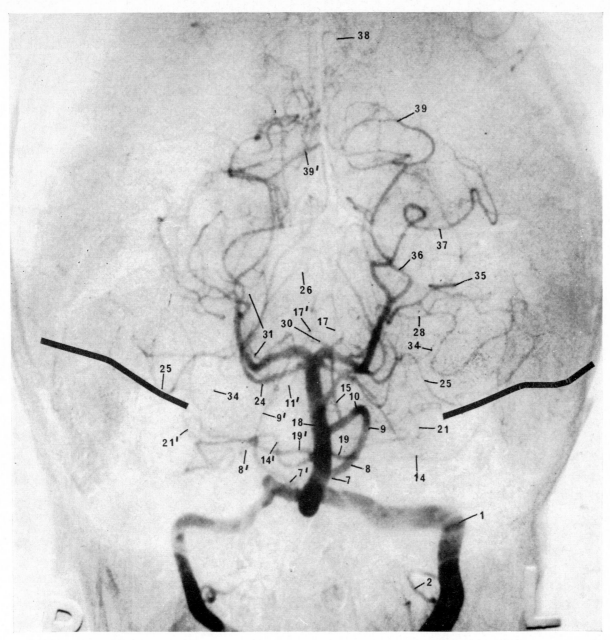

Figure 55

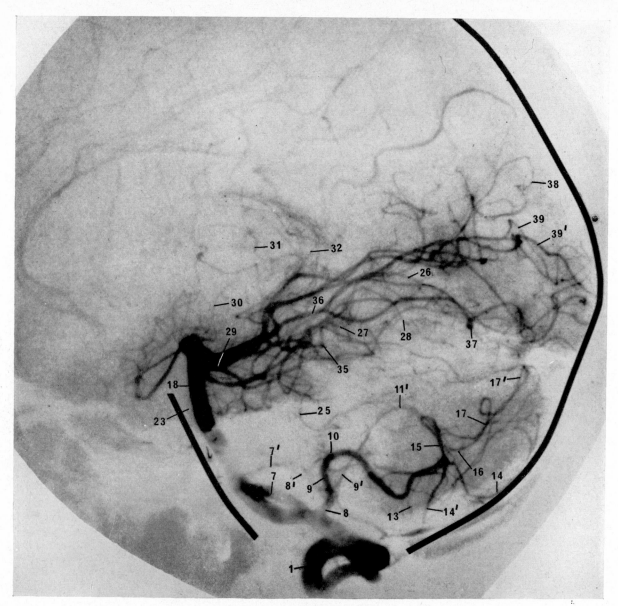

Figure 56

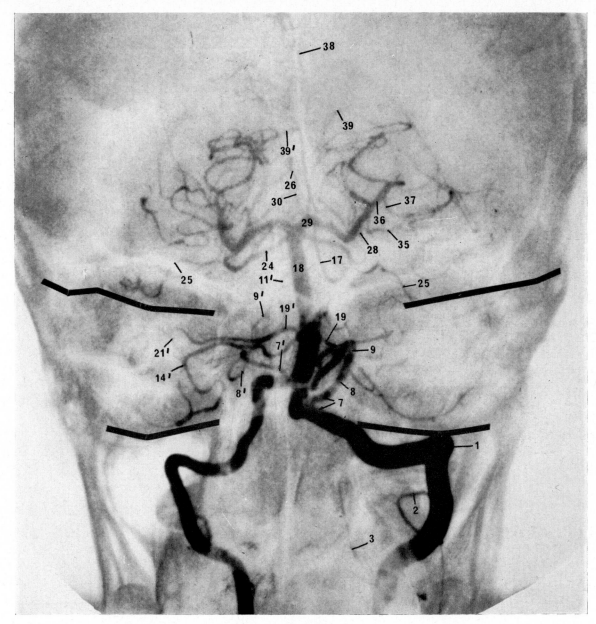

Figure 57

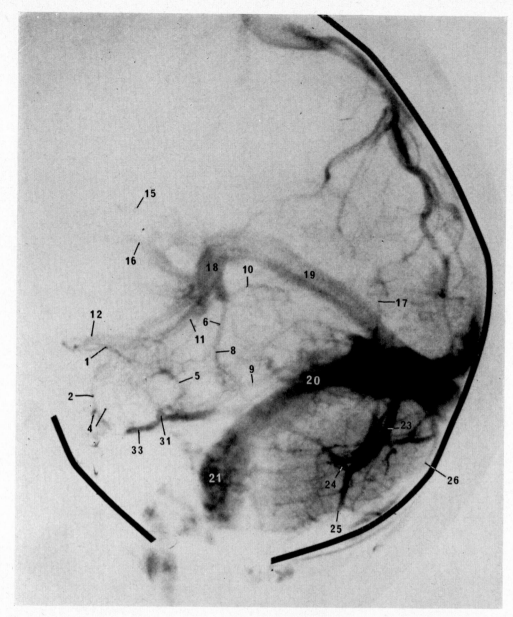

Figure 58

Case 11 (Figures 58–61)—*Venous system. Lateral, Towne's and antero-posterior views. The inferior vermian veins are unusually symmetrical and so are the hemispheric veins which, in the antero-posterior view, might be mistaken by the unwary for posterior mesencephalic veins.*

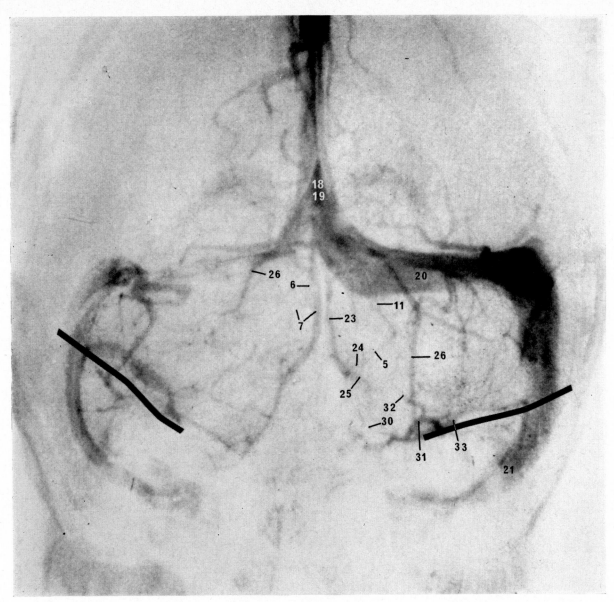

Figure 59

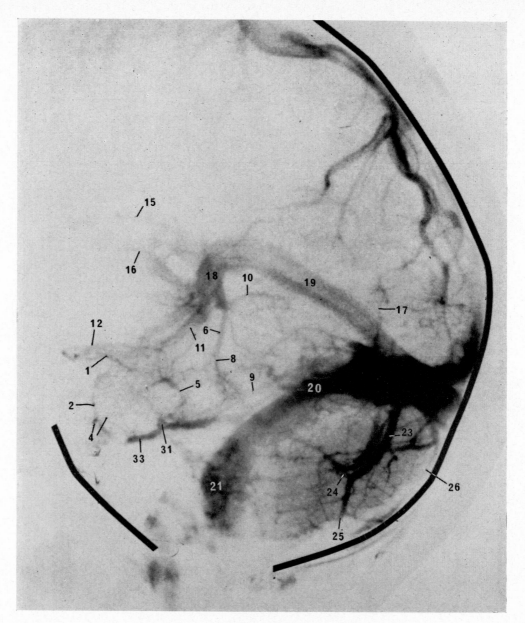

Figure 60

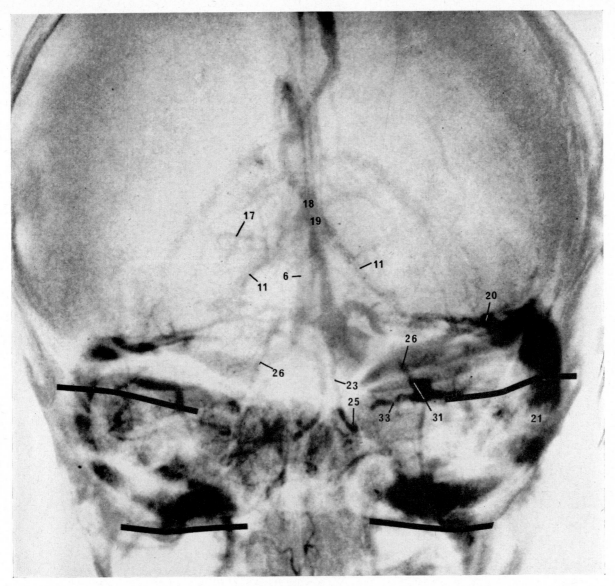

Figure 61

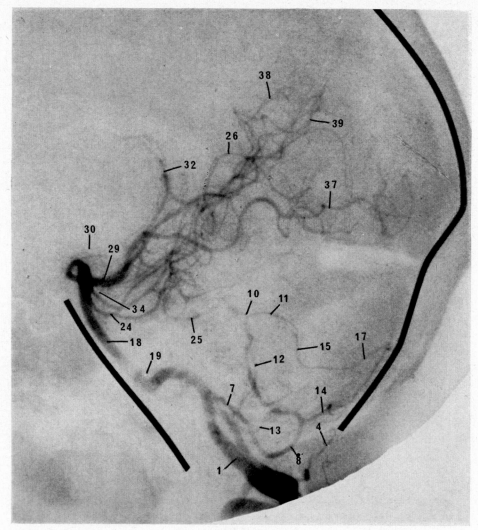

Figure 62

Case 12 (Figures 62 and 63)—*Arterial system. Lateral and Towne's views. The posterior meningeal artery is visible in both views. The anterior spinal can be seen in the Towne's projection.*

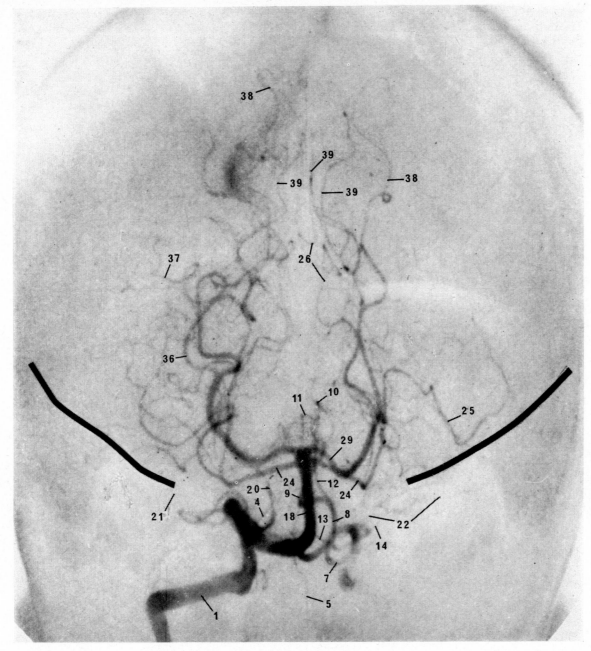

Figure 63

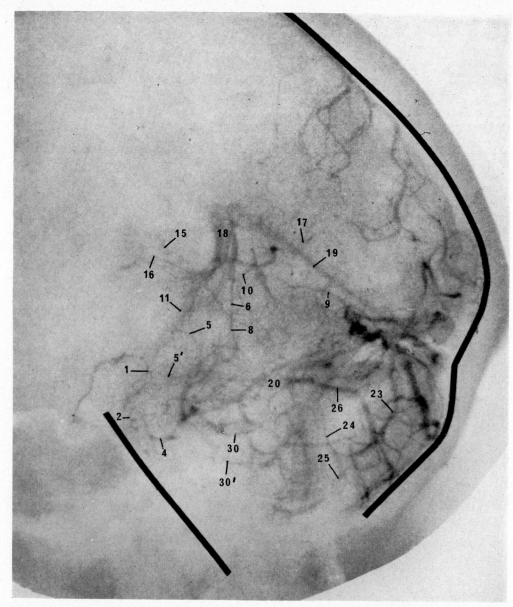

Figure 64

Case 12 (Figures 64 and 65)—Venous system. Lateral and Towne's views. The veins of the lateral recesses of the 4th ventricle are well shown. Notice their asymmetry.

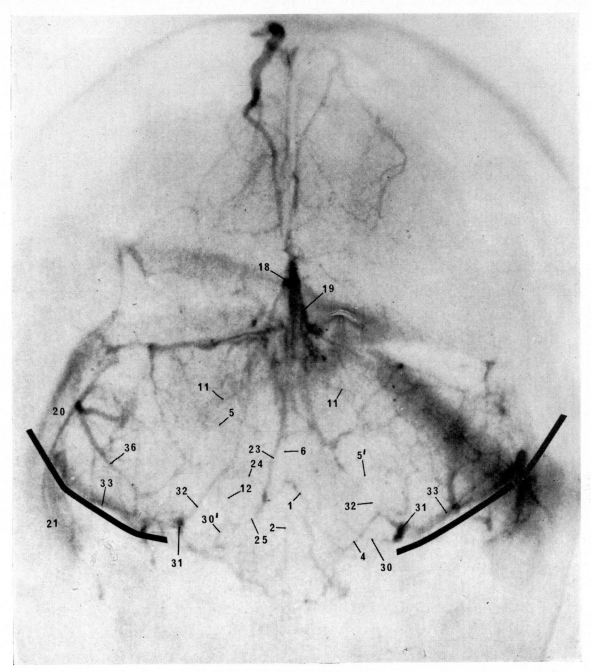

Figure 65

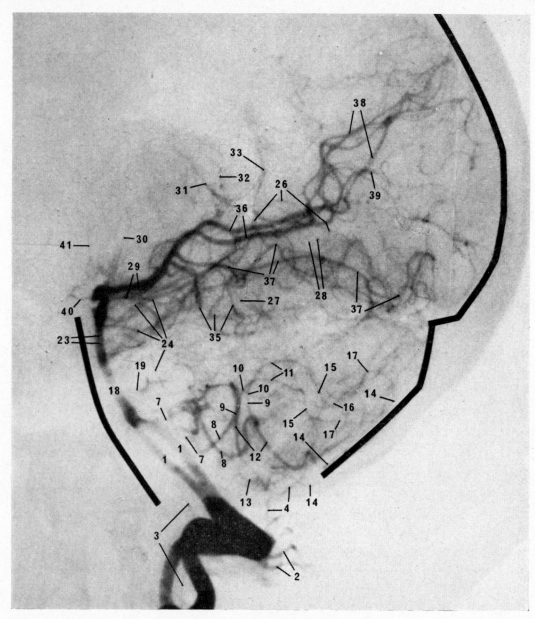

Figure 66

Case 13 (Figures 66 and 67)—Arterial system. Lateral and Towne's views. Both posterior inferior cerebellar arteries are filled, but they are so symmetrical that we have not been able to distinguish one from the other in the lateral view. The anterior meningeal artery is shown in the lateral view.

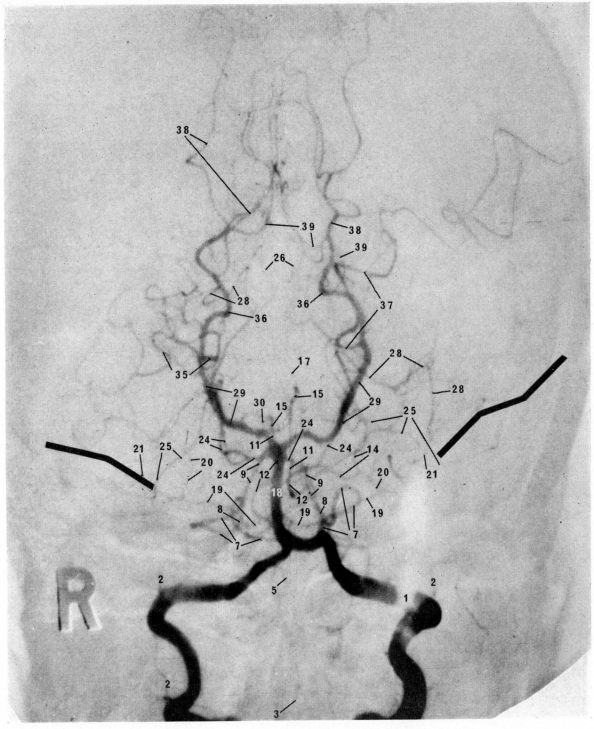

Figure 67

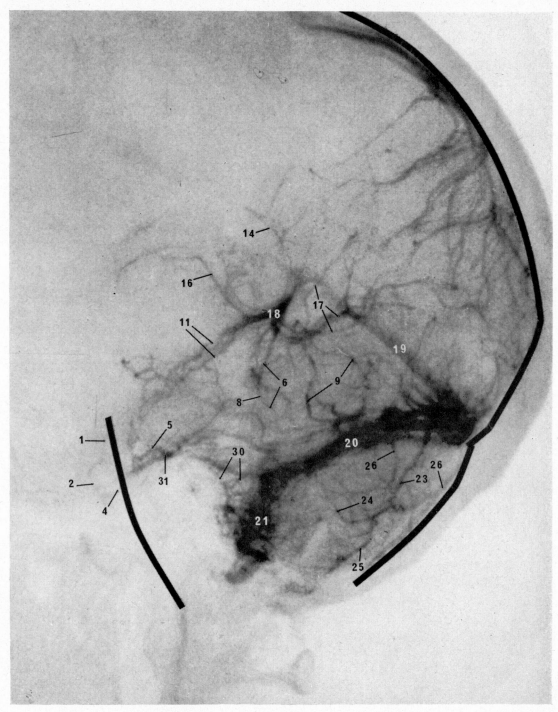

Figure 68

Case 13 (*Figures 68 and 69*)—*Venous system. Lateral and Towne's views. The peduncular tributary of the left posterior mesencephalic vein is clearly seen in the Towne's view.*

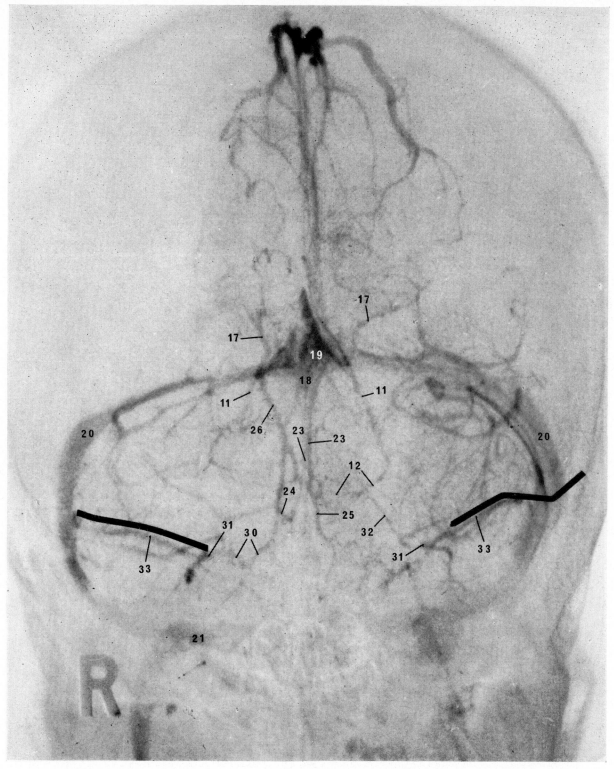

Figure 69

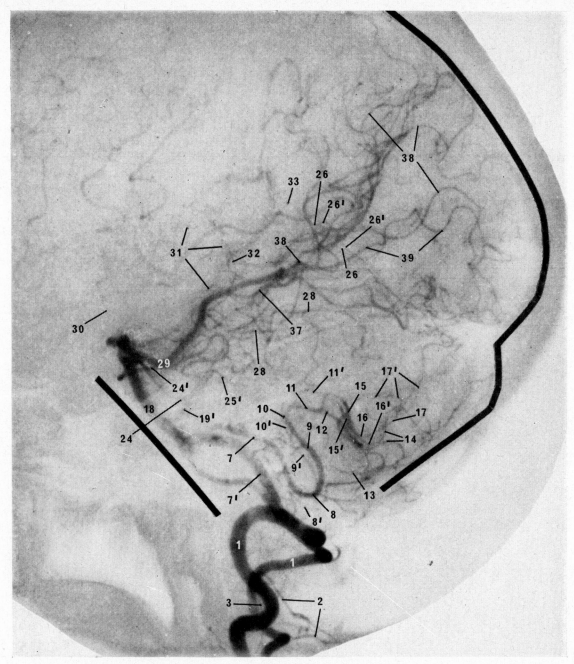

Figure 70

Case 14 (Figures 70–73)—*Arterial system. Lateral, Towne's and antero-posterior views. The vertebral arteries are of irregular calibre. In the antero-posterior view only one is filled and only one posterior inferior cerebellar artery outlined. In the other views both posterior inferior cerebellar arteries have been shown. The left, the larger, is distinctively labelled. An attempt has also been made in the lateral view to distinguish the right from the left superior cerebellar artery.*

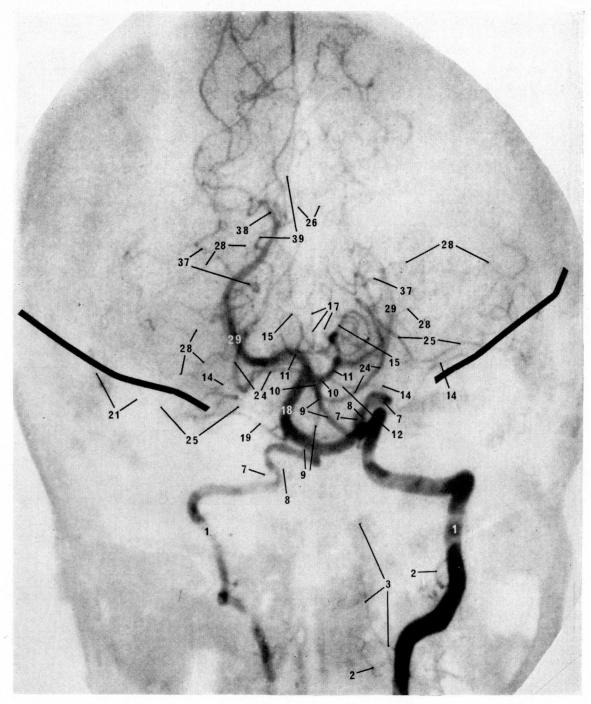

Figure 71

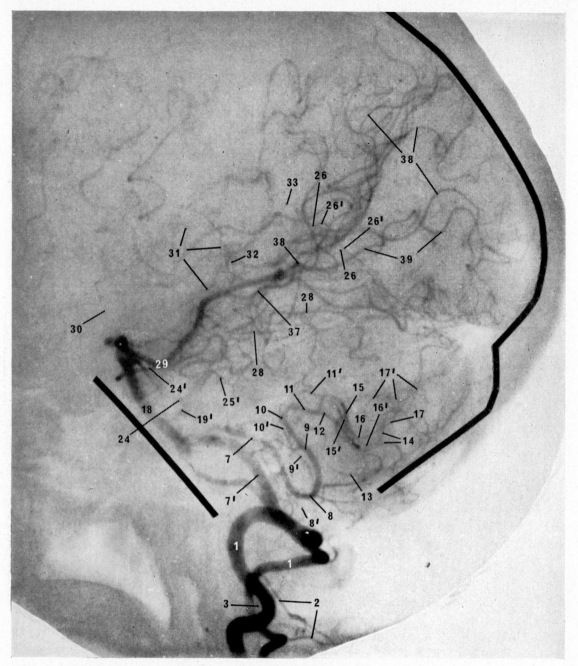

Figure 72

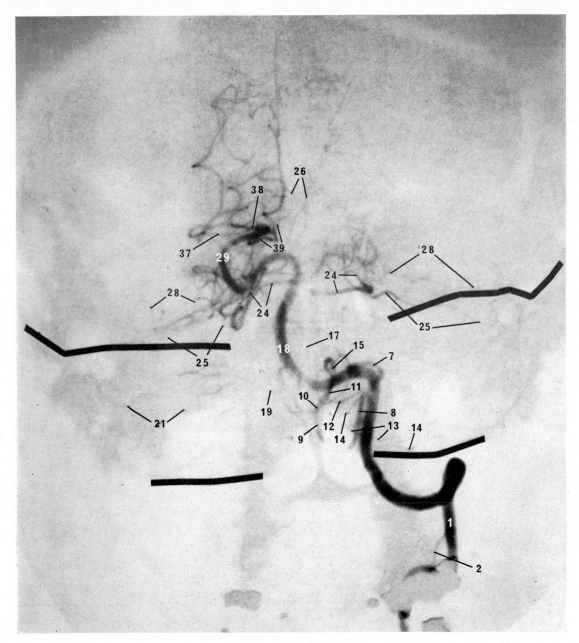

Figure 73

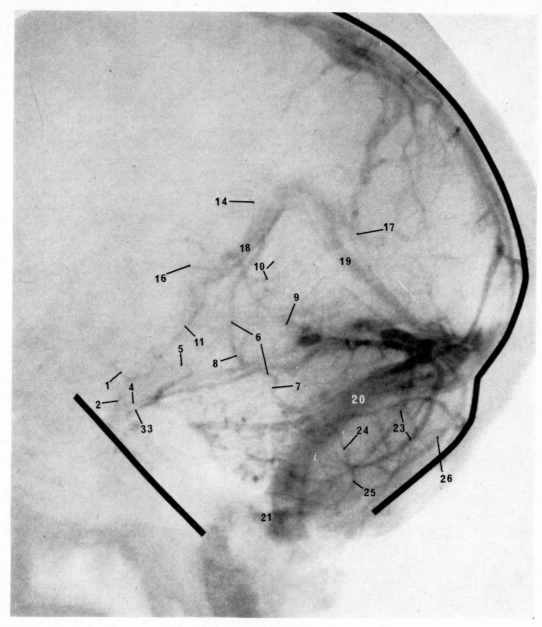

Figure 74

Case 14 (Figures 74 and 75)—Venous system. Lateral and Towne's views. The pontine segment of the anterior ponto-mesencephalic vein and the transverse pontine veins can be seen communicating in the Towne's view. The precentral cerebellar vein has a large brachial tributary in direct communication with the petrosal vein.

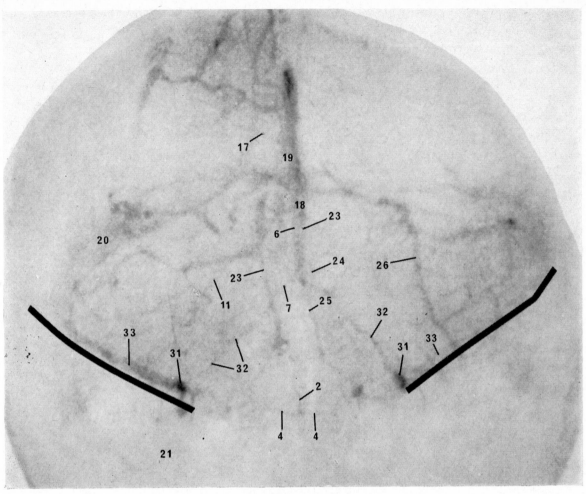

Figure 75

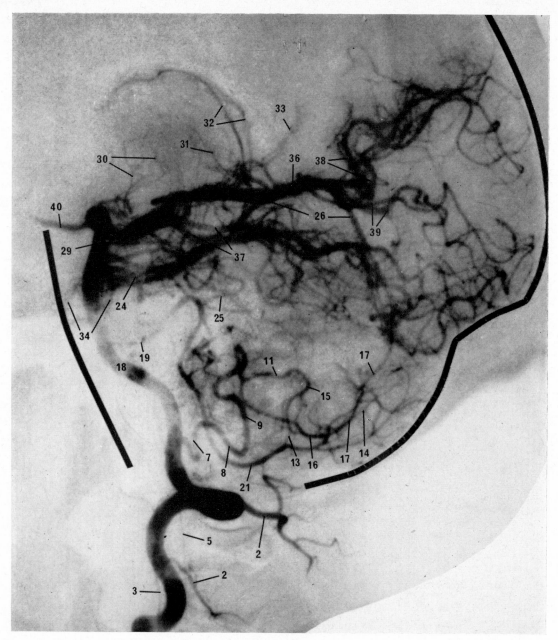

Figure 76

Case 15 (*Figures 76 and 77*)—*Arterial system. Lateral and Towne's views. Note that the right-sided tonsillo-hemispheric branch, shown in the Towne's view, must arise from the left posterior inferior cerebellar artery. The left anterior inferior cerebellar artery has an enormous lateral hemispheric branch which supplies a substantial part of the left cerebellar hemisphere. The anterior meningeal and the anterior spinal arteries are both visible.*

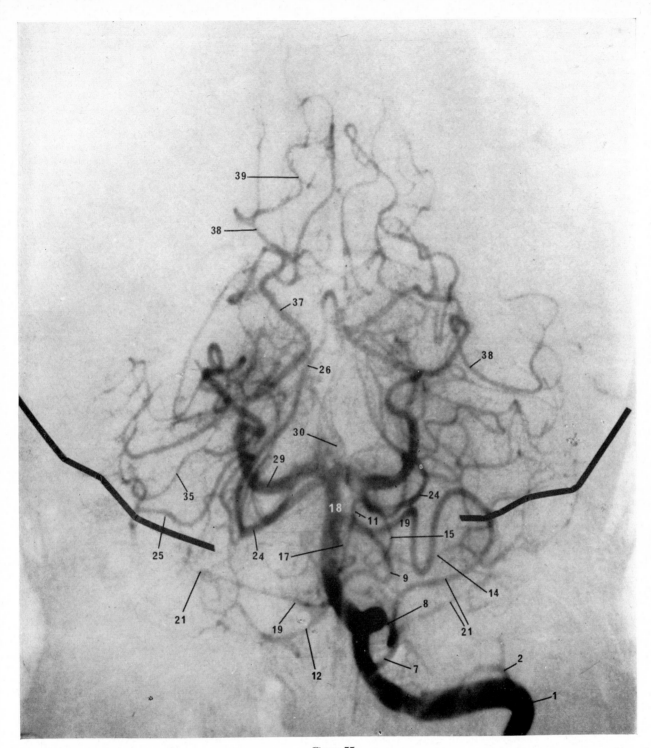

Figure 77

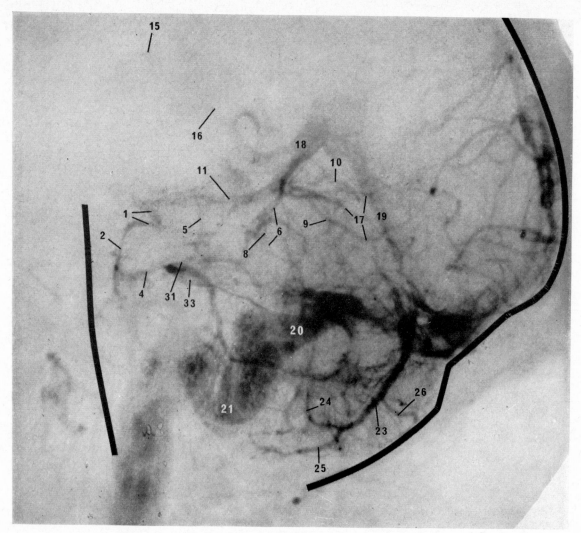

Figure 78

Case 15 (Figures 78 and 79)—*Venous system. Lateral and Towne's views. The large superior and inferior retrotonsillar tributaries of the inferior vermian vein are noteworthy. The superior choroidal and thalamic veins are both shown in the lateral view.*

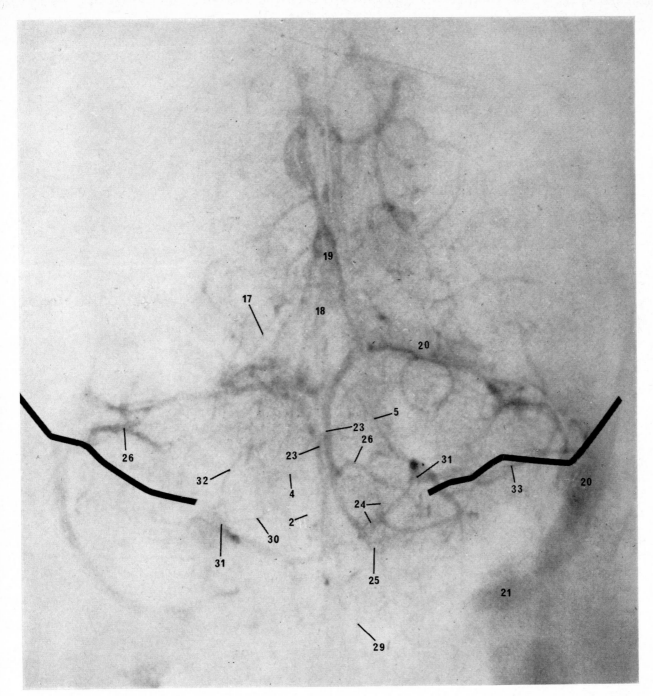

Figure 79

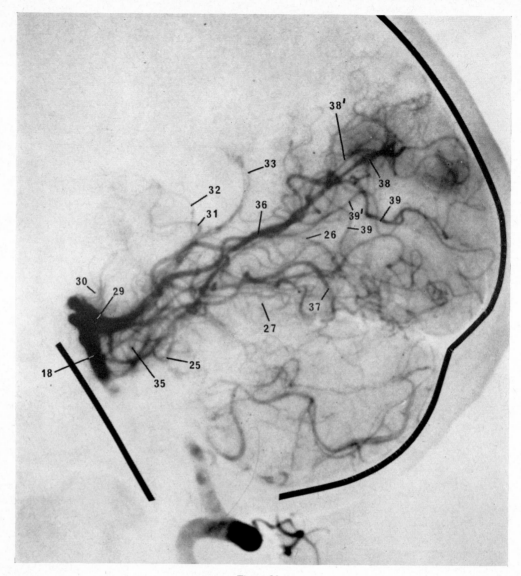

Figure 80

Case 16 (*Figures 80 and 81*)—*Arterial system. Lateral and Towne's views. Naming of the terminal branches of the posterior cerebral arteries presents some problems. It is probably correct to recognize two calcarine arteries on the left.*

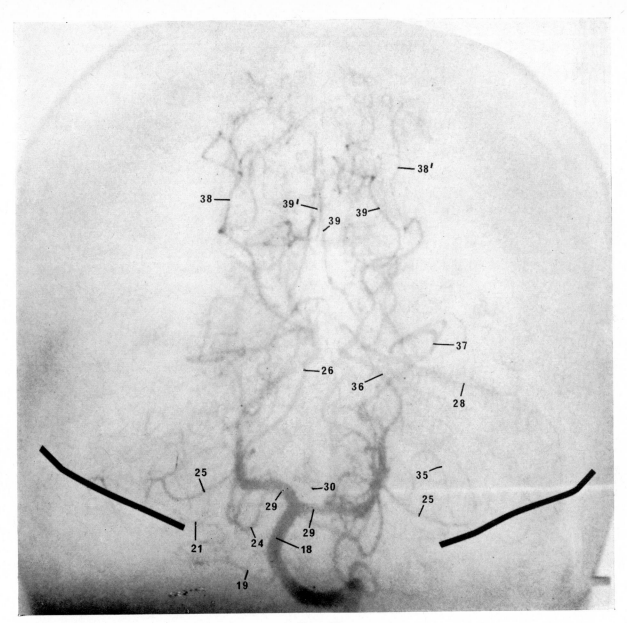

Figure 81

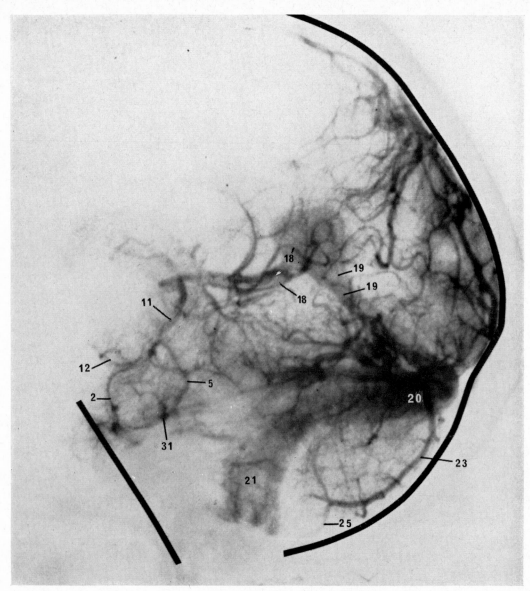

Figure 82

Case 16 (Figures 82 and 83)—Venous system. Lateral and antero-posterior views. There is a very large lateral mesencephalic vein. The anterior part of the posterior mesencephalic vein is missing. The anterior ponto-mesencephalic vein probably drains to the petrosal via a large transverse pontine vein.

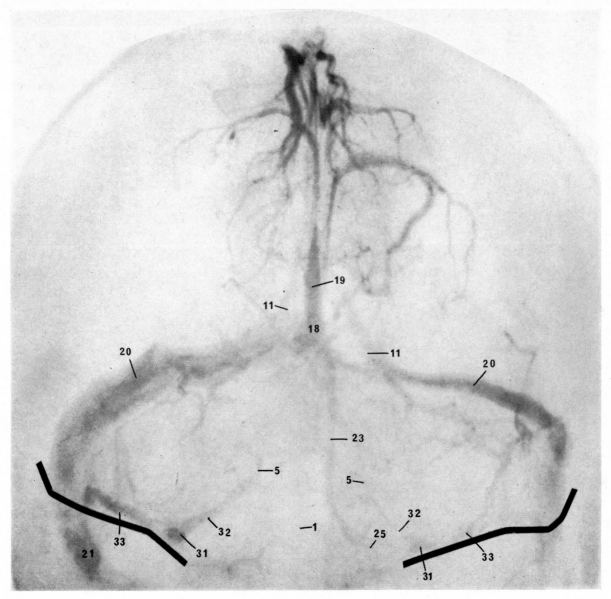

Figure 83

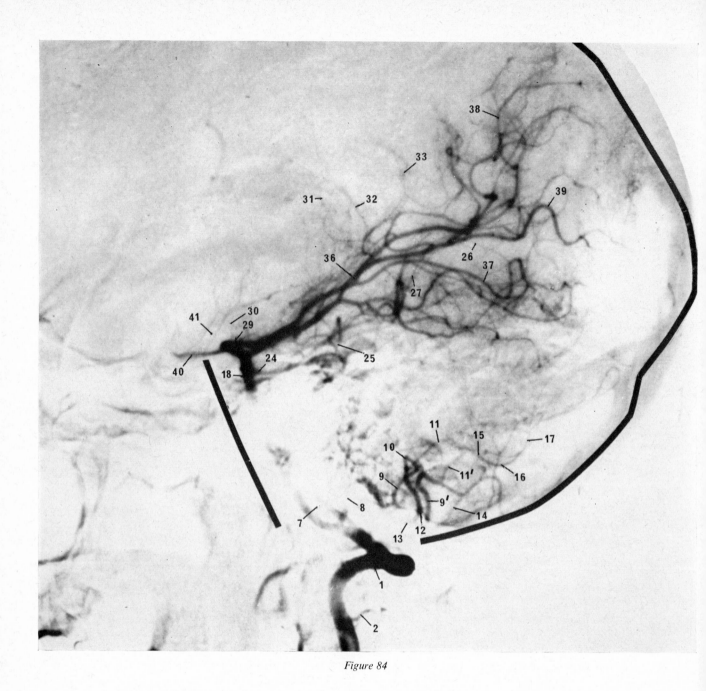

Figure 84

Case 17 (Figures 84–87)—*Arterial system. Lateral, Towne's and antero-posterior views. In the antero-posterior view only one posterior inferior cerebellar artery is shown, but in the Towne's and lateral views both have been filled and are separately labelled. This example shows the very common anomaly of two superior cerebellar arteries on each side.*

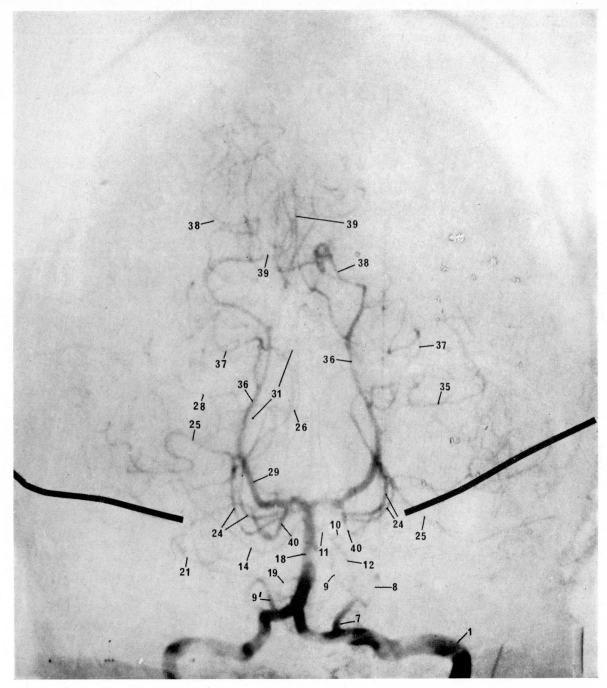

Figure 85

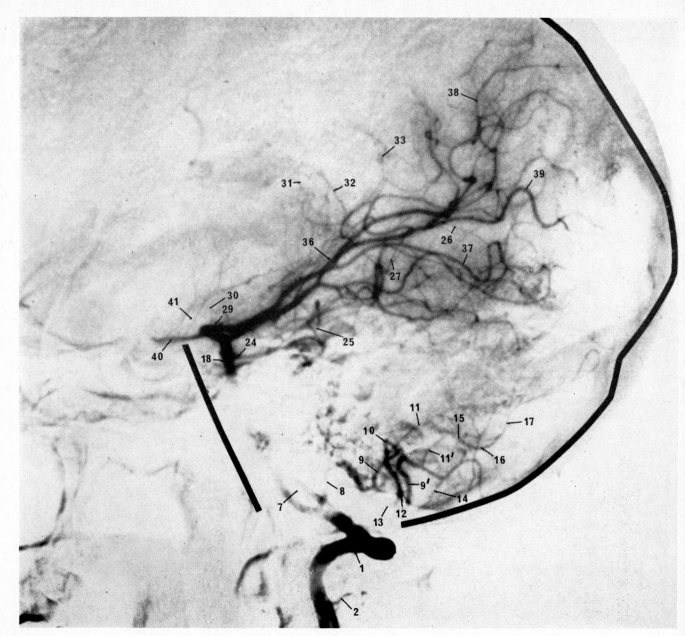

Figure 86

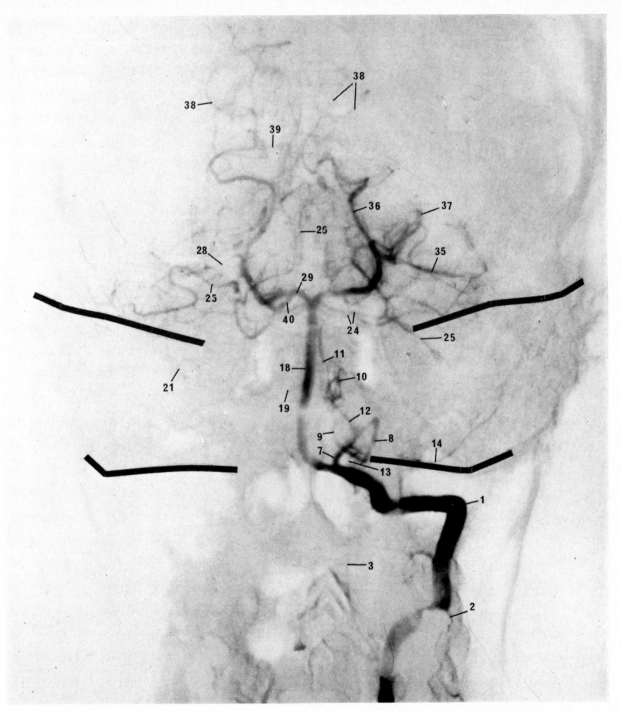

Figure 87

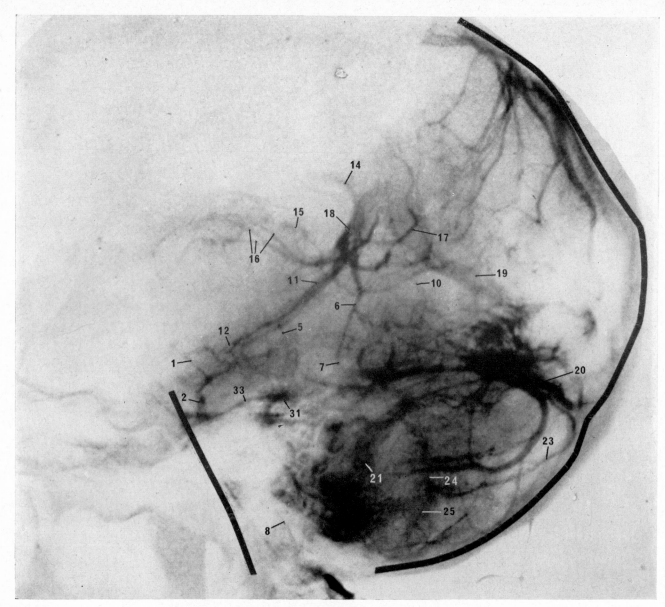

Figure 88

Case 17 (Figures 88 and 89)—Venous system. Lateral and Towne's views. The brachial tributaries of the precentral cerebellar vein communicate directly with the petrosal veins.

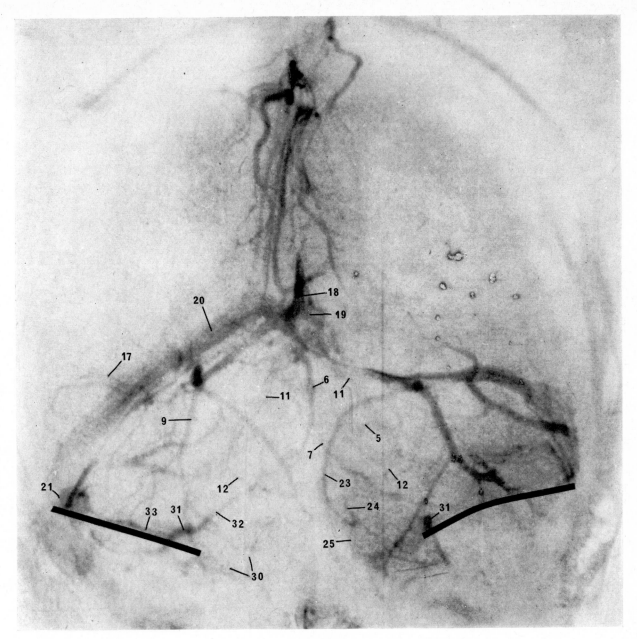

Figure 89

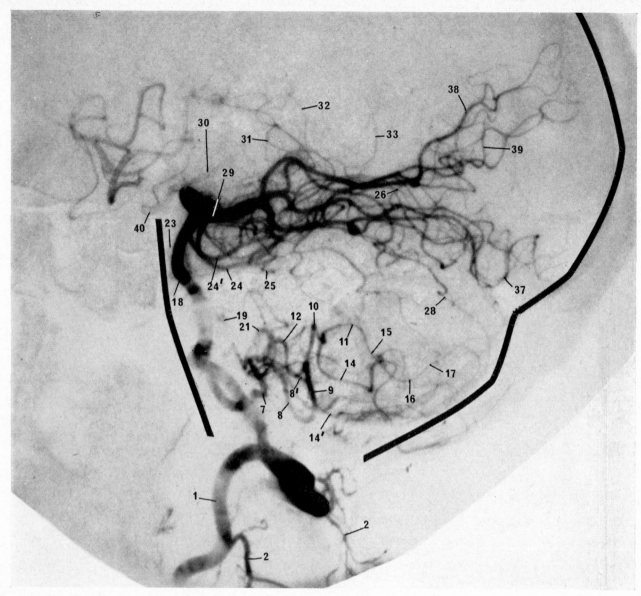

Figure 90

Case 18 (Figures 90–93)—*Arterial system. Lateral, Towne's and antero-posterior views. There is a strong possibility in this example that both posterior inferior cerebellar arteries arise by a single trunk from the left vertebral artery. The left anterior meningeal is filled, but has not been labelled.*

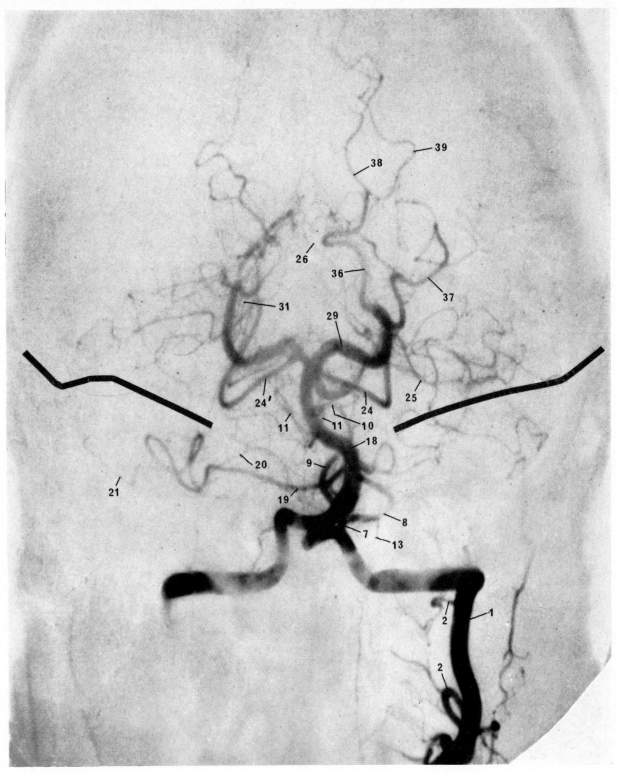

Figure 91

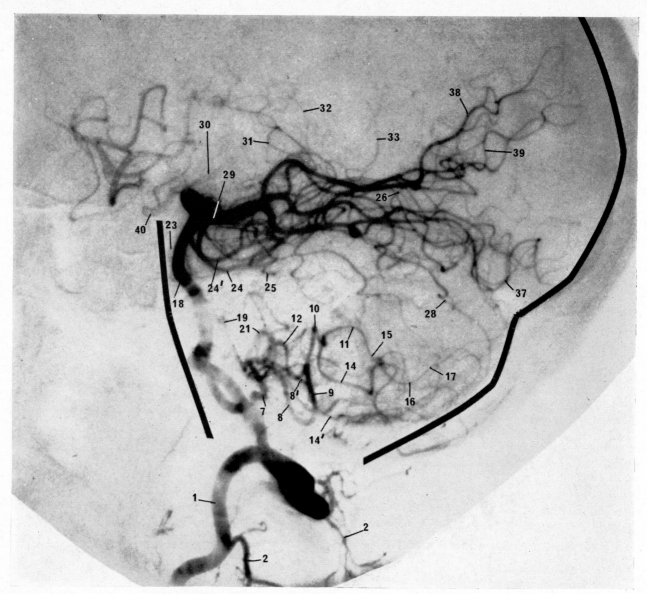

Figure 92

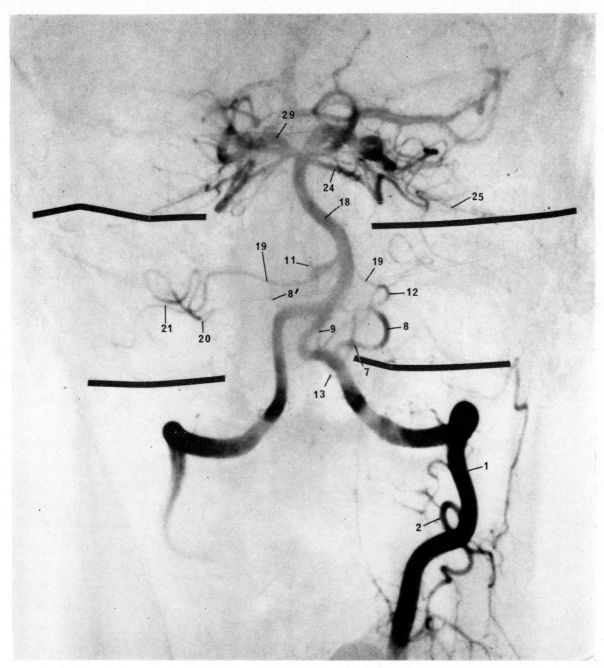

Figure 93

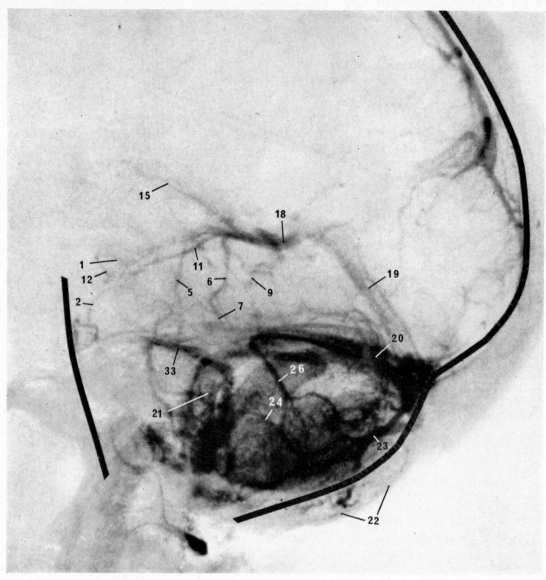

Figure 94

Case 18 (*Figures 94–97*)—*Venous system. Lateral, Towne's and antero-posterior views. The superior and inferior retrotonsillar tributaries of the left inferior vermian vein are well shown.*

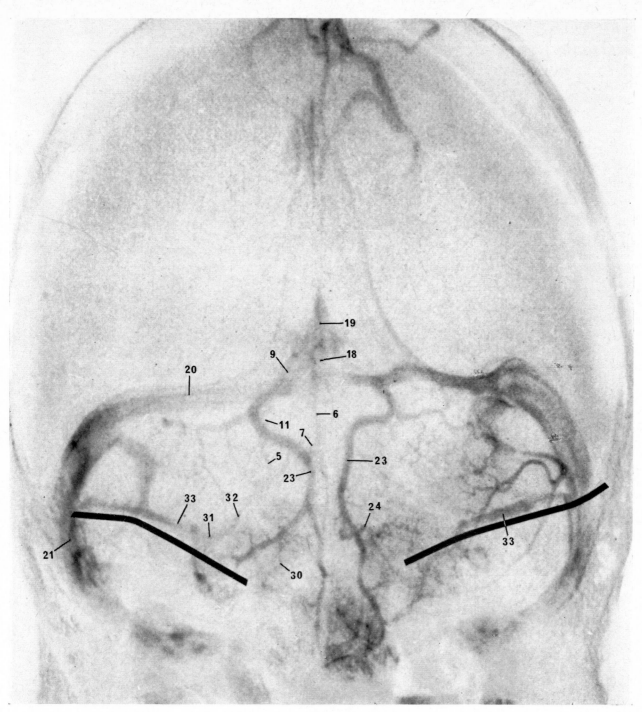

Figure 95

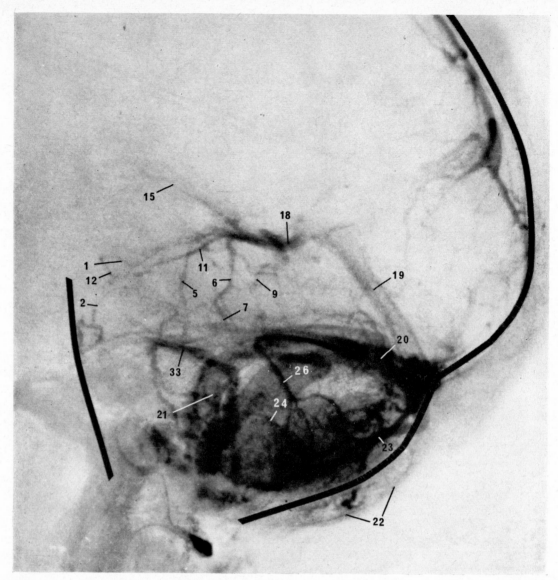

Figure 96

114

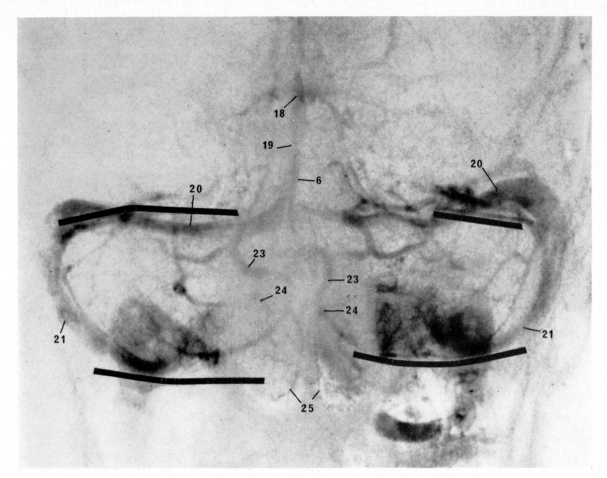

Figure 97

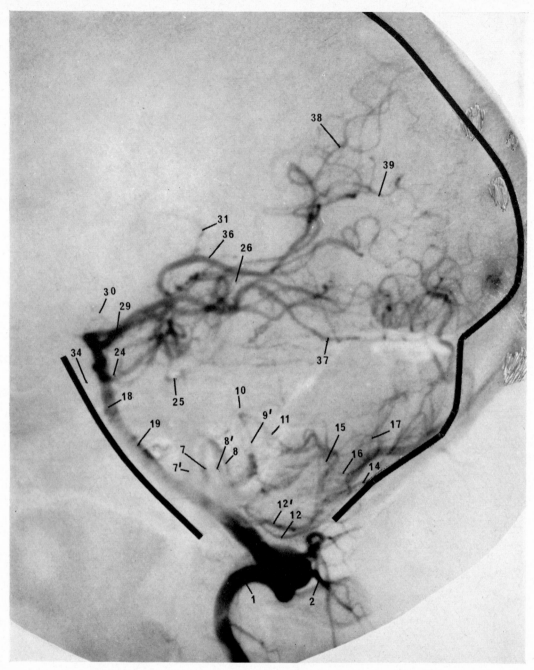

Figure 98

Case 19 (Figures 98 and 99)—Arterial system. Lateral and Towne's views. The two posterior inferior cerebellar arteries are separately labelled. There is a large communication between one of the muscular branches of the left vertebral artery and the occipital artery.

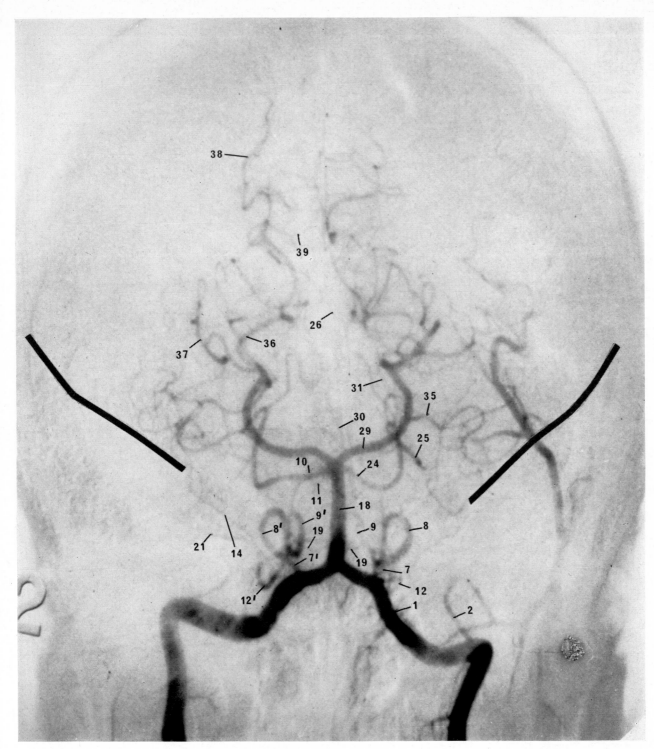

Figure 99

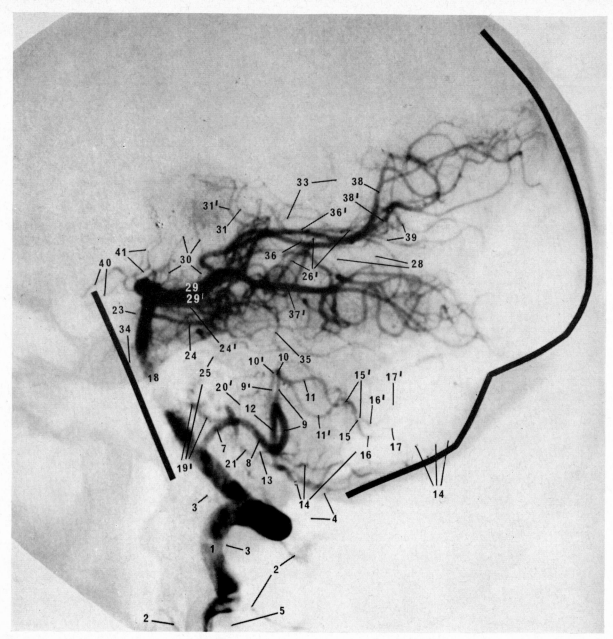

Figure 100

Case 20 (Figures 100-103)—Arterial system. Lateral, Towne's and antero-posterior views. The right vertebral is only a small vessel. The left is large and the basilar is its direct communication, swinging across the midline in a gentle curve. For this reason, the midline branches of the posterior inferior cerebellar artery are seen to the left of the main trunk of the basilar. Note the use of the antero-posterior view to show the tonsillar branch of the posterior inferior cerebellar artery and its relation to the foramen magnum, as well as a good right anterior inferior cerebellar artery. In the lateral view an attempt has been made to distinguish right- from left-sided arteries.

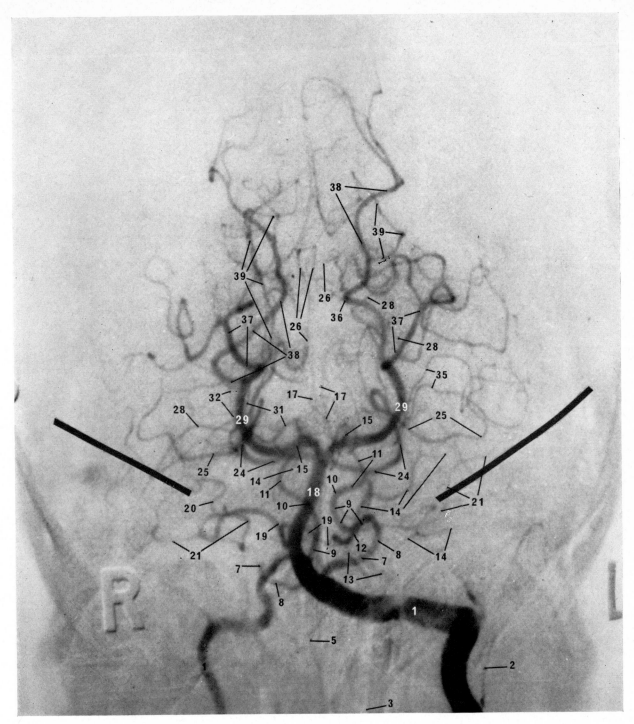

Figure 101

119

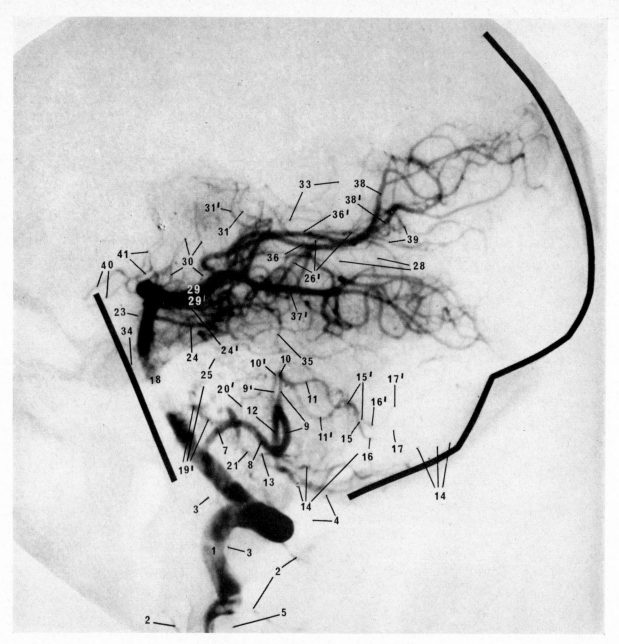

Figure 102

120

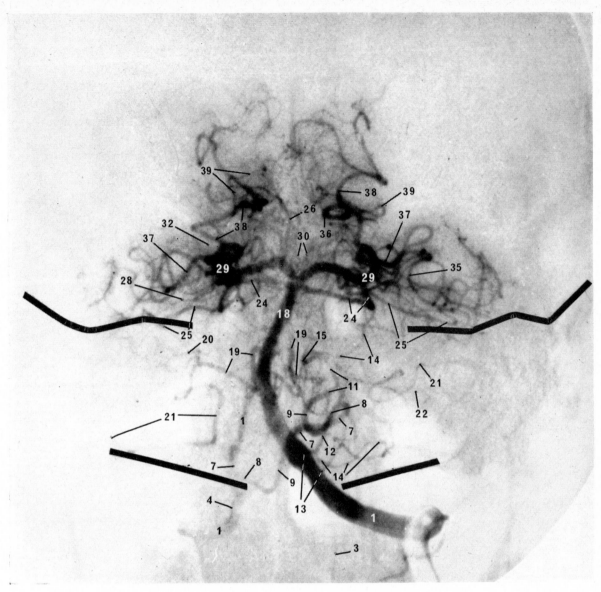

Figure 103

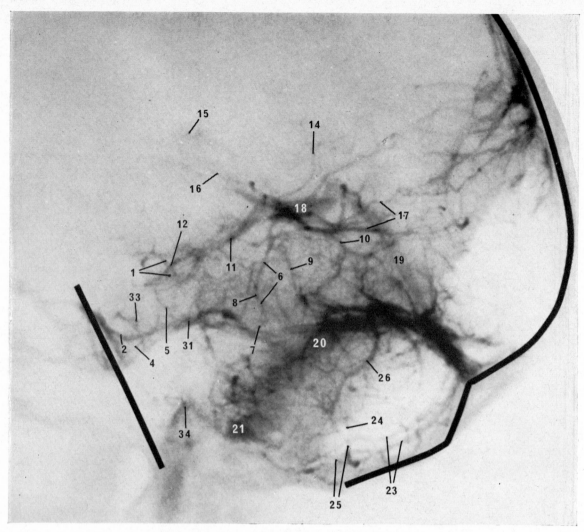

Figure 104

Case 20 (Figures 104 and 105)—*Venous system. Lateral and Towne's views. The precentral cerebellar vein is duplicated throughout its course. A very anteriorly placed lateral mesencephalic vein is seen in the lateral view, but does not correspond to the one labelled in the Towne's view.*

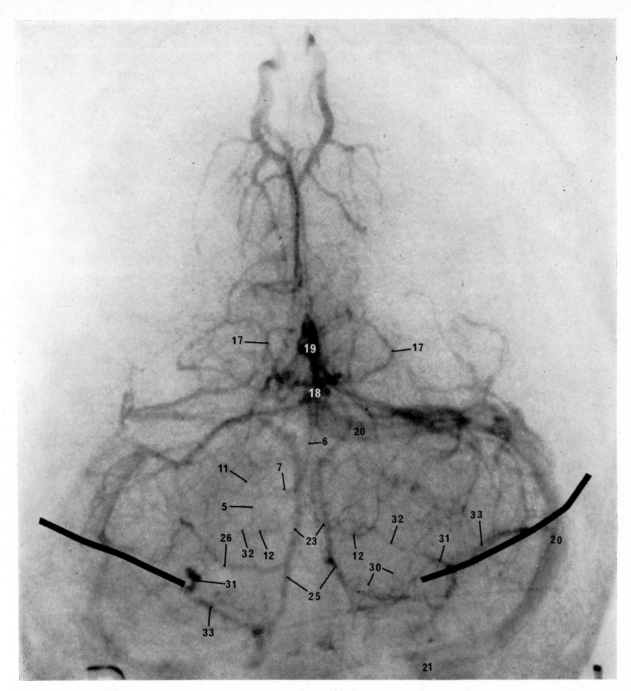

Figure 105

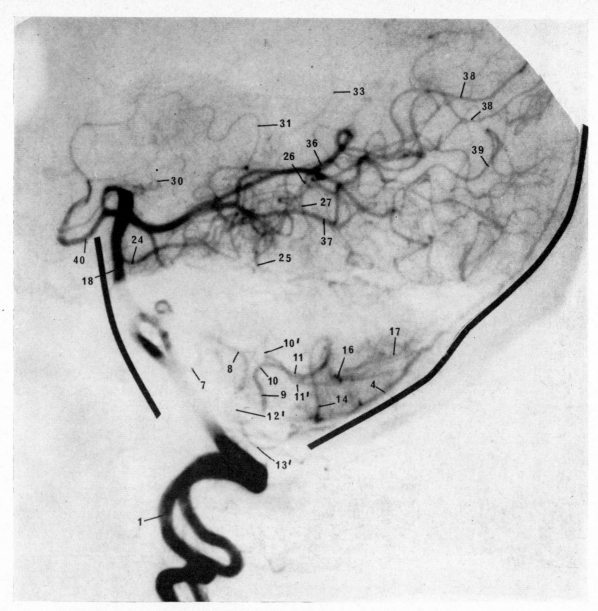

Figure 106

Case 21 (Figures 106 and 107)—*Arterial system. Lateral and Towne's views. There is a very large posterior meningeal artery. The right anterior inferior cerebellar artery gives rise to a tonsillo-hemispheric branch with a tonsillar continuation.*

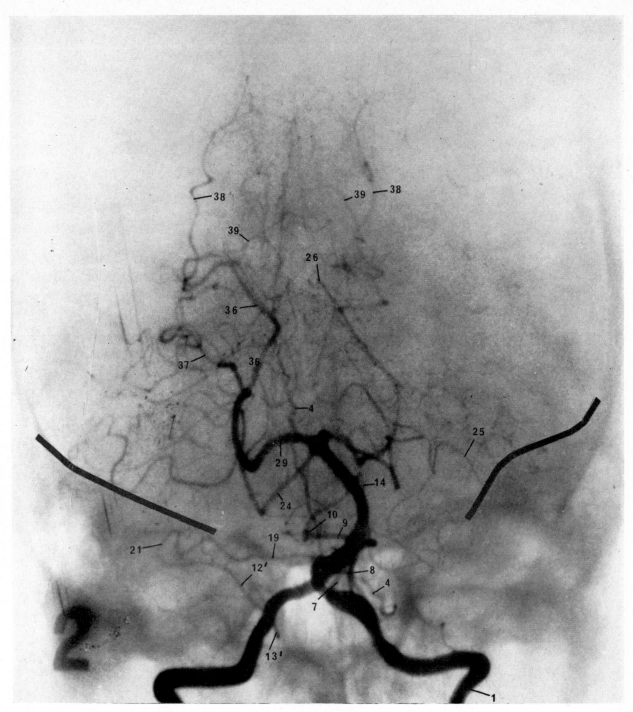

Figure 107

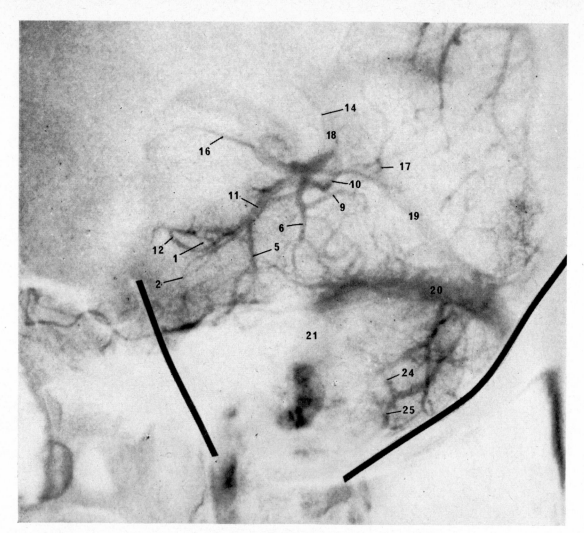

Figure 108

Case 22 (Figure 108)—Venous system. Lateral view. A particularly good example, showing one version of the relationships between the precentral cerebellar and the superior vermian veins.